BAL.

11/20.

THE SHIFT

THE SHIFT

*How I (lost and) found myself
after 40 – and you can too*

Sam Baker

CORONET

First published in Great Britain in 2020 by Coronet
An Imprint of Hodder & Stoughton
An Hachette UK company

1

Copyright © Sam Baker 2020

The right of Sam Baker to be identified as the Author of
the Work has been asserted by her in accordance with
the Copyright, Designs and Patents Act 1988.

A CIP catalogue record for this title is available from the British Library

Hardback ISBN 978 1 529 32976 6
Trade Paperback ISBN 978 1 529 32977 3
eBook ISBN 978 1 529 32979 7

Typeset in Miller Text by Hewer Text UK Ltd, Edinburgh
Printed and bound in Great Britain by Clays Ltd, Elcograf S.p.A.

Hodder & Stoughton policy is to use papers that are natural, renewable
and recyclable products and made from wood grown in sustainable
forests. The logging and manufacturing processes are expected to
conform to the environmental regulations of the country of origin.

For everyone who's had it with putting up and shutting up.

'The menopause comes, and it is the most wonderful fucking thing in the world. Yes, your entire pelvic floor crumbles and you get fucking hot and no one cares, and then ... you're free. No longer a slave, no longer a machine, with parts. You're just a person ... It's horrendous. But then it's magnificent.'

Kristin Scott Thomas in Fleabag

CONTENTS

INTRODUCTION

It dawned on me that something wasn't 'right' around the time I was 46. It could have been earlier, but after a lifetime of gynaecological chaos, I didn't pay much attention when my periods dribbled more or less to a halt.

My confidence crashed (not ideal when you've just ditched a high-profile job to start a business that depends, at least in part, on your capacity for self-belief and now you're standing in the kitchen howling that you're a failure and resigning was a terrible mistake). Where once I would have bulldozed straight on, confident on the outside, if not inside, now I simply couldn't see a way through. On top of that came the depression, which was less a matter of highs and lows than a case of lows and lowers. I had less than ever to 'be depressed about'; I just *was*.

Then came the sweats. Oh lord, the sweats. I'm not sure which was worse: the hot flushes during the day, when you could at least feel them roaring in and try to get to the nearest loo to lie down, body pressed to the cold (and inevitably vile) tiled floor until they passed. Or the night sweats. Often, I'd wake in a puddle, skin soaked, hair slicked to my body, sheet and duvet drenched. I seriously worried I'd started wetting the bed. WTAF was going on?

Then my good friend the flesh duvet moved in. And decided to stay. Indefinitely.

Of course, I had a suspicion, but I couldn't bear to accept it. I wasn't old enough. Was I? I was 46 going on ... I don't know, 30-ish. I looked young for my age, people always said. I *felt*

1

young. Wasn't menopause something that happened to ... old people? Was *I* old?

Despite the countless blogs and Facebook groups and, yes, self-help books, I didn't really know where to turn. None of my friends would admit to being perimenopausal yet, and seeking help on social media felt like a public admission of ageing. Which sounds ridiculous now, but then, only a few years ago, when no one would even whisper the word menopause, it felt like a huge deal. Eventually, unable to carry on in the body and brain of someone I hardly recognised, I barged into the office of the gynaecologist who'd helped me with my endless problems, yelling: 'HELP! GIVE ME ALL THE DRUGS!' Brushing aside her futile attempts to talk me through a leaflet explaining the link between HRT and breast cancer, I left triumphant with a prescription and the leaflet. I never did read it. Right then I didn't care about the potential risks or side effects. All I cared about was taking a 'magic pill' to bring me back to me. I took it. And, lucky for me, it worked. Slowly I started to re-emerge.

As months passed, I began to be able to identify other women with that faintly deranged WTF-is-happening-to-me look in their eyes, and a tendency to suddenly overheat. It didn't happen overnight. After all, it's not as if you can go up to complete strangers at parties and say: 'I noticed you look a bit hot ...' And at work I was surrounded by women up to 20 years younger than me. Their conversation was all about whether they would ever be able to afford to buy a flat and if/when to start trying for a baby. Why would they care about someone so ancient that their eggs – and plenty of other bits – were drying up?

If I'd known then what I know now, I would have approached the whole thing differently. I wouldn't have spent precious hours hunting down other women who looked a bit hot and irritable and kept tugging uncomfortably at their clothes. Instead, I would have developed a radar for the rare relaxed older woman you see – *very* occasionally – in the street, in cafés, at work dos. Rumour has it they are more plentiful in certain parts of America, but in the UK you have to look pretty hard to spot them. And, on finding them, I would have begged them to share their wisdom. How did they get there and what was it like on the other side? How did they shift from hot, flabby, depressed, confused and convinced they had early onset dementia, to calm, radiant and in control, with an indefinable air of togetherness and an ability to rise above the whole shit-show?

Journalists tend to romanticise or demonise menopause. It's a time when you supposedly either stop caring about the shape of your jeans and start wafting contentedly along beaches in wide-legged linen trousers, sensible sandals and floppy hats, or become the plate-smashing heroine of Revenge of the Menopausal Woman. Unsurprisingly, the reality is not a lot like that. You're either judged for taking HRT or judged for not taking it, for 'giving up' or living in denial, for Botoxing or not Botoxing. The list of things you're doing wrong is endless. And, let's face it, that list was never short. Just ask a pregnant woman. (Or indeed any woman.) Plus everyone is suddenly an expert – especially the berks on the internet – but in reality nobody knows enough about the menopause. And that includes the bulk of the medical profession.

But don't despair! This book is here to show you that on the other side of menopause there is a whole new life and an opportunity to discover a new, unexpected version of you: a body, mind, attitude and sexuality that is recognisably you but different. A you who is not ruled by your fertility – or lack of it.

It's called The Shift.

The Shift from living a life spent contorting yourself into shapes that accommodate the male gaze, to being in the happy position of being ignored by it. And you know what? You won't care.

The Shift from your place in the world being assigned solely on your youth and beauty, as it is for young women, to being able to

3

decide what *you* want that place to be. Because – guess what? The patriarchy is no longer paying attention to you. You're no longer interesting. The eye of Mordor has moved on, and so shall you.

The Shift from being a person (OK, a woman) who is constantly asked about and judged on their ability to have children (whether or not you have or want them), to being just a person: you, but without the oestrogen, and consequently a lot more attitude, confidence and, quite possibly, rage. Quite a bit of rage TBH. Because if there's one thing menopause gifts you, it's a righteous fury; an indignation and a staunch inability to suffer fools, injustice and inequalities. As Angela Davis, author of *Women, Race and Class*, puts it: 'I'm no longer accepting the things I cannot change. I'm changing the things I cannot accept.'

This book is about The Shift from having your narrative laid out for you by society – husband, babies, house, then what? – to becoming storyless. Or, as I prefer, story-free. There is no preordained story for women after Happy Ever After. (After all, according to the history books – clue's in the 'his' – we're meant to have a baby or five, then die and be replaced.) But when The Shift comes, we're free to write our own. And that's where the fun kicks in. When nobody's looking, it means there are fewer boundaries preventing you from doing cool shit and getting things done.

Because let's be honest, the problem is *not* you. You're fine. You're better than fine. You're on fire. (Possibly, quite literally.)

The problem is a society that sees a woman who, no longer childbearing, has 'outlived her usefulness' and doesn't really know what to do with her. In fact, it doesn't really *see* us at all. It's an advertising industry that thinks all women are under 40 (in fact, make that thin, white, able-bodied, cis-gender and straight)and it doesn't seem to be remotely interested in taking your money if you're not. What a bank-balance-boosting trick it's missing. It's a fashion industry that cuts clothes for teenage girls and doesn't acknowledge that women of 40, 50, 60 and beyond might still want to look like themselves even if it does take a bit more work – and better-quality fabric – to pull it together. It's a beauty industry that only cares about flogging us anti-ageing products and hair dye so we can pretend we aren't 50, and a media industry that thinks a once-a-year anti-ageing issue is all it takes to keep us happy (or at least quiet). It's a business environment that treats men in their fifties as if they are in their prime and women in their fifties as if they're past it. It's a world where, frankly, men are solidifying and women are being disappeared. It's time we took a leaf out of the millennial handbook and stopped putting up with it. It's time we grasped that invisibility society has bestowed on us and saw it for the blessing it can be.

So if you're feeling sidelined, invisibled, ignored. By the media, the advertising industry, the fashion industry and waiters and bar staff the world over. If you've been talked round and over and asked to take the minutes or make the tea too many times to mention. And, worse, have put up with it. This book is for you. And it's for me – seven years ago, hot, angry, confused, anxious and desperately seeking solidarity. *The Shift* is the book I wish had existed when I didn't know where to turn. The book to show me life wasn't ending but beginning.

If you're in the vicinity of 40, you might not have noticed The Shift looming on your horizon yet. If you're in your mid-/late forties, you probably have an inkling of what's to come. A sense of trepidation. Or, like I was, you could already be in the throes of it. Chucked in at the deep end without a clue. Fifty and beyond? You know exactly what I'm talking about. Let's take a step back and look at this objectively, shall we?

- **We have power.** (Trust me, we do! It just might not always feel like it). So what if you're 'bossy' or 'aggressive' or 'difficult' or all those other things women have always been accused of? It's called knowing your mind and standing up for yourself.

Get used to it. And, in the immortal words of almost every woman ever, 'I love it when they underestimate me.' Because while they're not paying attention, you can cause trouble and be disruptive right under their noses, in a way that you never could when you were paying rent in 'their world' with your youth and beauty.

- **We have freedom.** Those who had children are beginning to regain their freedom and those who didn't, or couldn't, no longer have to endure lengthy phone calls from their mothers asking when they're going to give her a grandchild. The shackles of societal expectations when it comes to 'what makes a woman' and what a woman should do in her life are falling away. Don't cling on to them. You don't need them.

- **We have money.** For many of us, this will be the first time in decades we have disposable(ish) income to spend how we want. If we're lucky, we can work fuller than full-time if we want; we can cut back and spend the rest of the time doing our own thing; or we can retrain. We have adaptable skill sets that we can use any way we choose; and we can do it all without having to worry about who's paying for childcare.

- **And, contrary to received wisdom, we have more guts, confidence and energy than ever.** We've lived a life and more. We've had our hearts broken; we've had abortions and miscarriages and struggled to conceive; some of us have experienced childbirth, others have lived through judgement in the face of the decision not to; we've been bereaved and we've grieved; we've survived health scares – some of them life-threatening; we've been pulled apart and we've put ourselves back together again; we've lost jobs, loves, homes and lives. But we're still standing. We're strong. We're resilient. We know more than ever. Now it's time to channel it.

- **And, you know what? Many of us have reached a point where we simply don't give a fuck. (Or know how to identify the worthless fucks at least.)** We've spent our lives in boxes, trying not to touch the sides, scared of what might happen if we do. But you know what happens? Nothing. The walls are just constructs, built by the feeble hands of the pale, male and stale. The boxes will collapse. We are bigger than the box – if only we realise we're allowed to be. We know what works, we know what suits us, we know who and what we are. We are slowly, surely, starting to care less. As Gwyneth Paltrow said in *The Sunday Times Style*, 'You're no longer A/B testing all your behaviour and all your stuff out there in the world, because you're done, you don't give a f***, you're like, "This is me."'

The Shift is not a guidebook or a handbook, or a step-by-step medical guide to menopause. Or even a book about menopause per se. Plenty of those already exist and I'm not a doctor or health expert. I can't tell you exactly what vitamins to take or which fabrics best absorb sweat or whether or not you should take HRT. I don't have all the answers – or even some of them. I can only tell you what happened to me, a woman who stumbled into perimenopause without a clue what was coming for her, and with an existential dread that the end was nigh.

What I discovered in the seven years it took me to get from first(ish) hot flush to that one momentous menopausal day (when I hadn't had a period for a year and bells ring and birds sing and people buy you cake and flowers and white wine no longer makes you feel nauseous. Just kidding!) was that menopause isn't an abyss, it's a bridge – to something new and unexpectedly exciting. If only someone had told me sooner. So I'm telling you now. Perimenopause can be shit (gotta be honest, mine was) but after the shit comes the shift – which is why this book is divided into two halves: imaginatively titled The Shit and The Shift. I've covered everything I experienced and more, as frankly as possible. Possibly a little too frankly in places. You might notice there's no single chapter about mental health. That's because – it turns out – the whole book is about mental health. It's perimenopause's big secret, the thing nobody tells you: along with the sweats and the physical and sexual changes, it will wreak havoc in your head. But it will also give you the opportunity to re-evaluate everything as you emerge on the other side. Or maybe that's just me.

And that's the other thing. Because there are as many experiences of shifting as there are of being a woman, and I didn't want this all to be about me and the limited experience of a straight, white, cisgender woman, who was born working class but has spent most of her adult life working in the media, I recruited over 50 women from all backgrounds, mainly via social media, and canvassed them on every subject at every stage along the way. They come from a variety of races, classes and sexual persuasions, their ages range from 40 to 70 and they are at various stages of perimenopause, menopause and post-menopause. (I've included their ages, not because I approve of women being judged by their age, but because I thought it might be useful for you to be able to compare their experiences with your own.) They are ordinary women from ordinary backgrounds and you'll find their stories scattered through these pages. I hope you'll get to know them a bit, as I have. All we had in common when we came together was that we were all fully sick of the shitty end of the stick that's thrust at women over 45. We all wanted to do something about it, so we started by talking honestly, candidly and, so, sometimes, for some of them, anonymously. Those women have been the biggest gift of writing *The Shift*: those funny, smart, angry, lively, sweary women. Women I didn't even know existed a year ago are now women who've shared their deepest secrets.

The Shift is for those women, and women like them; women like me and you. Women who are not about to put up and shut up. It's time we harnessed our crazy, chaotic, creative, collaborative power and wrote ourselves a new narrative. We are the most underestimated and ignored demographic in society (cheers, the patriarchy). Well screw that. Because to be a woman in your forties/fifties/sixties and beyond in the 21st century is to be a force to be reckoned with.

Part One:

THE SHIT

'Perimenopause and menopause should be treated as the rites of passage that they are. If not celebrated then at least accepted and acknowledged and honoured.'

Gillian Anderson

1

FUCK ME, I'M BOILING

From hot flushes to brain fog and chronic, incapacitating anxiety; the symptoms you know to expect – and the symptoms you very much don't

'Give me all the drugs!'

I swear, those are the first words I utter when I surge into the gynaecologist's office, wild-eyed and sodden. Stripping off as many layers as I decently can, I fling my bags on the floor and myself into the just-comfortable-enough-but-not-so-comfortable-you'll-stay-too-long chair facing the chaotic desk of my overworked saviour.

'I'm serious.' I flap my shirt, feeling warm, damp air sort of circulate around my clammy boobs. 'Just give me the drugs. *Please*.'

The gynaecologist, Claire – a woman now in her mid-fifties who has spent more than her fair share of time looking at my uterus over the past decade or so – smiles knowingly and mirrors my movements, tugging at the neck of her top in a vain attempt to let the air in or, perhaps, the heat out. She's in the same overheated, over-crowded boat, she tells me, she's just been in it a couple of years longer. Then she opens the dog-eared cardboard file on her desk that contains the history and mystery of my vulva and extracts a pre-printed sheet of paper.

Even through the blur and the heat and the exhaustion, I know I'm luckier than most. Rather than doing battle with whichever GP I can luck into an appointment with four weeks next Thursday, I am able to go straight to someone who knows me inside and out. She knows I bleed often and by the bucketful – until a few months ago, when my periods stopped altogether. (Hallelujah!) She knows I'm not a massive drug taker. Apart from Ibuprofen. And Lemsip. Buckets of Lemsip. Oh, and the hardcore iron tablets I've taken daily since I started passing out – most notably on a side road off Oxford Circus – and my GP told me I was chronically anaemic, not because of massive monthly blood loss caused by what I later discovered were fibroids and polyps, but because I had been vegetarian-ish since I was 20. (I'd like to say the GP was a middle-aged white man, because I do like to pin as much on them as possible, but it wasn't, it was a young woman I'd specifically asked to see, thinking I'd get more empathy ...) I didn't even last that long on the contraceptive pill. So, I've never been super-keen to take more hormones. Plus, I am a fully paid-up member of The Sisterhood – or so I thought – and The Sisterhood, in the main, is of the opinion that HRT (hormone replacement therapy) is A Bad Thing. Not only a bad thing, but dangerous. And traitorous. And, worst of all, PLAYING INTO THE HANDS OF THE PATRIARCHY. Oh, and vain. And shallow. And ... I'm a feminist BUT give me HRT and give it to me now!

I'm not going to give you a science lesson (there are many far better equipped than me to do that). But for those of you lucky enough not to be in the know, HRT typically contains oestrogen (most commonly estradiol) and a synthetic progestogen to replace the hormones our bodies stop producing during perimenopause. Some women take a combined pill, some use oestrogen gel and take a progestogen tablet, others wear a patch. The options alone would take an entire chapter to sum up, but in a nutshell HRT, and its many permutations, has been in the eye of a medical and moral storm ever since it launched as Premarin in America in 1942 and was famously made from mares' urine. Aside from the extremely sexist taglines used in its advertising until recently (here's a sample: *He Is Suffering From Oestrogen Deficiency, Is She The Reason Why?*), many studies published over the last two decades have connected it to increased risk of breast cancer, particularly in older women taking it upwards of five years. There is also believed to be a slight risk of ovarian cancer.[1] On the flipside, women who take HRT in whatever form are found to be less likely to develop osteoporosis and urinary tract infections. And that's before you get started on the moral and political issues. Of which there are MANY.

I'll go into it more later, but all you need to know is that, at this point, I don't give a damn about any of it. I don't care which side thinks I'm letting them down. I don't care if I look weak or vain or in denial or insufficiently stoic. I don't give a rat's arse what I'm putting into my body. And I'm not interested in the much-publicised health risks – although the flaky wind of publicity changes constantly. Tell me if you must, I think, but *na-na-na-na-nah I'm not listening*. I see your increased breast cancer risk and I raise you osteoporosis and the chronic state of my mental health. (I didn't say I was being responsible, I said I was desperate.) I am hot, I am often drenched, I am anxious – fearful even. I am sleepless, I am forgetful, I am confused. I am alternately enraged and hollowed out, empty. I am given to uncontrollable outbursts of temper and equally unpredictable floods of tears. In the kitchen. In the office loos. On the tube. At home, in the shower, where – bliss! – no one can see you howl. My self-belief is at rock bottom and I am even more of a confidence-free zone than usual. I have totally lost sight of myself. I do not know who I am any more. (And that's before I get started on the hair loss and weight gain.) All this would be bad enough if I was still doing the job I have done successfully for over 20 years. But, no. In my wisdom I chucked that in and am now 'self-employed' and in the early days of starting a business.

In this, as with all the other things on this list, I am not alone. I know that now. Utter confusion and lack of awareness seem to go hand in hand. But I didn't know that then; then, I thought I was going mad. So mad, in fact, that more than once (OK, more than ten times) I googled 'early onset dementia'. I wasn't alone in that either. About 10 per cent of the women I interviewed were so convinced they were showing early signs of dementia that they actually went to the doctor. More than 50 per cent considered it.

Anyway, I have tried everything I can think of and I am all out of options. In short, I am desperate.

'Please,' I repeat, slightly calmer now. 'Give me some HRT. I just want to feel like me again.'

Claire hands me the sheet of paper and gives me her 'this is important' stare as she talks me through the pros and cons; the links between HRT and an increased risk of breast and uterine cancer in older women, and the health benefits (yes there are some, starting with reduced incidence of osteoporosis and UTIs). I nod and make appropriate uh-huh noises. As soon as I decently can, I shove the leaflet in my bag with a fingers-crossed promise that I will definitely, positively, honestly, read it thoroughly later. NOW give me the drugs.

This is the point I should stop and scroll back, because this is not the beginning. Far from it. It's the end of the beginning. Or maybe it's the beginning of the middle. Either way, I'm on the cusp of a resolution, of sorts, and I need to tell you how I got here: clammy and hysterical (sorry, but hysterical *is* the right word in this case) three floors above Harley Street, about to willingly drop 350 quid I don't have. Let's start where *it* started, roughly 18 months earlier. *It* being perimenopause, something I knew very little about until it smacked me in the ovaries. I'd heard about the sweats – all you ever hear about are the sweats – but the sweats are the tip of the iceberg. For me, at least, the other symptoms were far more debilitating. If I had known *those* symptoms were perimenopause and not that I was seriously losing my grip, I'd have sought professional advice a lot sooner.

See? Already we're in a place of confusion – a place that will become familiar to you if you spend any time at all thinking about or talking about or indeed experiencing perimenopause. Because even though sweats are the symptom most commonly associated with perimenopause, what even are they? Are we talking about sweats or are we talking about hot flushes – or hot flashes, as Americans call them? Are they the same thing, or are they perceptibly different? I wish I could tell you. All I know is what I experienced. And, chances are, your experience will be different. The main thing I've learnt from the dozens of women I spoke to for this book is that there are as many experiences of menopause as there are women – some good, some bad, some horrific, some brief, some lengthy, some still ongoing decades later (I know!), some ... neither here nor there. Everyone is unique and every one counts because afterwards you emerge different, changed. Shifted. In my case, dramatically. And for the better.

Back to me and the flushes/flashes/sweats. For the sake of argument, I'm going to split them into two groups: 1. night sweats, for the waking in the middle of the night in a puddle with your pjs stuck up your bum like you wet the bed and your hair clinging to your neck and your pillow turned to a sponge. Inconvenient, uncomfortable, insomnia-inducing, relationship-stressing, yes, but not publicly humiliating. 2. hot flushes/flashes, for the daytime onslaught that roars in from nowhere, usually when you're in the middle of an important meeting, making your temperature soar, drenching your clothes and, if you're really lucky, turning your face, neck and chest bright red. For me they were more like flashes – coming in from nowhere, rather than rising up from my core as many women describe. (A friend of mine suffered from these so badly that her assistant learnt to spot them and took to yelling, 'tropical storm incoming!' to give her a chance to escape to the loo to regroup. It's one way of coping, I suppose.)

I don't know how long I'd been having night sweats before I realised I wasn't just 'getting a bit hot'. They started gradually. First once a week, maybe twice. Then most nights. Then almost all night. In an attempt to regulate my temperature without actually throwing the duvet on and off at regular intervals, I developed a habit of sleeping with one leg hanging out of the bed, even in winter, where previously I had been a winter-thickness 13.5 tog duvet and two blankets kind of girl. In a (failed) attempt not to wake my husband Jon with constant duvet-tossing, I briefly experimented with 3am wanders down to the kitchen to ram as much of my body as I could get into the fridge. But the cat just thought it meant he was due a pre-breakfast snack and woke Jon anyway, so that was the end of that. Instead I would wake somewhere around two or three, damp sheets clinging to my skin, and start to pull apart the previous day, taking issue with everything I had said and done – or not done. What did X think of me? Why did Y respond like that? Why did I make that decision? Why didn't I? Then I would slowly drift back to sleep, brain cells still worrying away at my many perceived failings, only for another sweat to come lapping in and the whole process to start again.

All night, every night.

When the alarm finally went off at 6.30am – what felt like seconds after the last sweat – I was panic-stricken and exhausted.

If I was sensible I'd have kept a diary, but I'm not and I didn't, so I don't know whether this pattern of intermittent insomnia had been going on weeks or months when the daytime flashes began. I feel like a bit of an idiot typing that. Just as I feel like an idiot saying I didn't at first realise what was happening to me. From where I'm sitting now – safely on the other side and bloody glad to be here – it's so blindingly obvious. What I was thinking? *Was* I thinking? Probably not. My brain was fried from catastrophising all night and trudging through fog most of the day. But in my defence, I was only 46, and while perimenopause at 46 isn't unheard of, it's definitely on the early side. None of my friends were experiencing anything like this – or so I discovered when I plucked up the courage to ask.

Also, I'd bought into the whole idea that gets peddled by a certain section of the media that I could expect to have broadly the same menopausal experience as my mum. (God knows why, since, to my knowledge, gynaecologically we have little in common.) So I asked her. 'Mid-fifties I think,' she said vaguely, like it had been no big deal. And who knows if it had been or not, because like many women of her generation, she probably either thought it was something you didn't talk about or just got on with it, or both. An opinion she voiced – as did the boomer mothers of most of the women I spoke to. An unspoken, 'So why can't *you* just get on with it?' left hanging in the air. (As Lisa, 52, put it: 'In the immortal words of my mother, "I was fine. I just had to get on with it." Thanks, Mum.') So, I patted myself on the back and congratulated myself on having the great good fortune not to have to worry about menopause for another ten years. I certainly didn't put the sweat and the heat and the increasing amount of time spent lying on the grim-but-cool tiled loo floors at work together and make three.

(Handy tip: if you are, in fact, reading this lying on a public toilet floor praying for a flash to subside, don't. It's very very germy. Instead keep a can of Diet Coke – or fat Coke, entirely up to you – in the nearest fridge. Don't drink it. Just get it out of the fridge and shove it up your jumper. It's way more hygienic. Oh, and always carry a spare pair of knickers. Lots and lots of spare knickers.)

One whole year, almost two, of feeling unpredictably, unmanageably physically and emotionally out of control. Like there's someone driving your body, doing wheelies and handbrake turns (one of the women I spoke to somewhat randomly called her menopausal interloper Jane: 'My middle name – because I felt plain, invisible and cried at everything') and somewhere, trapped inside, there's you.

So, in a weird way, while the sweats are the least of it, they are the crux of it, too. The chicken and the egg. Or the no eggs. (Sorry.) While they can feel pretty much impossible to control (give or take cutting back on alcohol. Do as I say, not as I do ...) they are the thing you're primed to expect, even if you don't know how to deal with them. For me, all the rest came spiralling out of them. You sweat and overheat, therefore you can't sleep, you can't sleep therefore you worry, you worry therefore your anxiety levels go through the roof. When you do finally sleep it's time to wake up, so you start the day emotionally and physically drained, which in no way helps with the confusion, lack of confidence and anxiety you already feel. Then the flashes kick in. Try doing that on repeat for the next several hundred days while holding down a job, managing a team, looking after a family, maintaining a relationship (if you're heterosexual, with someone who's never going to go through it and as likely as not doesn't get it; if you're not then quite possibly with someone who's also living through it right now. Either way, is it really a shock that so many relation-ships break up right around now?). And remaining vaguely human while you do it. It's like being 15 but with all the responsi-bilities of a 50-year-old. Which is, after all, what it is: all the hormonal upheaval of puberty but in reverse. I'm not proud to say I failed to pull off either puberty or perimenopause with any degree of grace. It's only down to the extreme tolerance of my partner that I'm still married at all.

With hindsight, it's painfully obvious what was going on. But I was chronically unprepared for the massive life shift that was coming for me. Menopause stands alone in that regard. Look how open we are about periods, and pregnancy. Thanks, in large part, to millennial women who are zero tolerance on pretending to be 'just like a man' and keeping their premenstrual cramps and

PMS under wraps, we talk and talk and talk some more. At the water cooler, in the coffee shop, in the toilets at work, on email, on the office Slack, on WhatsApp groups, on Zoom. We know who's having their period, who's got cramps, who suffers from endometriosis and has to work from home once or twice a month, and who has medically chronic PMS. We diarise when to expect it for our own protection as much as anything else. But even as a teenager in the 1980s at my woefully inadequate comprehensive that thought showing us a film in biology of frogs fucking did the job when it came to explaining the intricacies of heterosexual intercourse, and anything else was TMI, I knew what to expect when my periods came and what the hell they were. for. I can't speak personally from a pregnancy perspective, but you can't spend 30 years working in offices full of thirtysomething women and not learn something.

But menopause ... not so much.

Imagine how great it would be if, just as we share our stories of massive blood loss and gut-shearing cramps, we compared sweats, brain fog and random crockery throwing, painful sex and debilitating anxiety, in the coffee shop queue. Despite the prolif-eration of blogs and Facebook groups, that still feels quite a long way off.

In part this is because menopause is the undeniable proof that we are ageing. We are NOT YOUNG ANY MORE (that's emphasis, by the way, not menopausal shouty caps). And God forbid we admit that, let alone celebrate what comes next. (Menopause shower, anyone?) And yet, all around, women of roughly my age are dying. But we're still here, still going, still being and doing and achieving, albeit with a few more wrinkles. WTF are we moaning about?

That's not to say the whole thing might not be a lot more bear-able if we knew a) broadly what to expect and b) that while menopause inevitably represents the end of womanhood as we are trained to know and value it – our biologically 'useful' years *gags* – what lies beyond can be equally, if not more, rewarding. That there *is* life at the end of this long, dark, hot tunnel. That's part of it, for sure. But the other part is that we simply don't know enough about it. And how scandalous, how enraging, is that? It's only going to happen to every single one of us, after all. That's just under 51 per cent of the global population at the last count.

I'm going to say this now and apologise in advance because I can absolutely guarantee it won't be the last time I do, but imagine for a moment this, THIS happening to the other 50 per cent of the population – the 50 per cent that is actually 49.2 per cent, if we're being picky. This thing shrouded in confusion and mixed messages, strong yet frequently ill-informed opinions, contradiction and lashings of shame. And they (the 49 per cent) are expected to just 'put up with it'. And, so, they do? Nah, me neither. But like I said, plenty of time to rant about that later.

Under-informed as I was, it eventually dawned on me what was going on, through a chink in the brain fog, or 'pink fog' as it was dubbed in a small study carried out by Miriam Weber in 2013.[2] (Why is it always pink?) It was the sweats that ultimately gave it away. But even with the certain knowledge that I needed to get myself some information and some support and fast, I couldn't really bear to accept it. I was 46. To borrow a phrase from journalist Kate Spicer, who tells me she doesn't mind being 50 but she's 'not ready to stop looking in the mirror', I 'presented' as youthful. I dressed youthful. I'd never overdone it on the tanning front (ginger, freckles, prickly heat, no choice) and a lifetime spent working in women's magazines meant I'd been on the receiving end of an awful lot of free moisturiser. I have zero belief in its miracle-conjuring properties, but applied twice a day every day for 30 years it has to have done something. Above all, I *felt* young-ish. Or I had. Was I now old?

(The short answer, of course, is yep. *Older* anyway. Nothing wrong with that. But that's the point, isn't it? To be a woman in the 21st century – a so-called first-world one anyway – is to be irrationally terrified of ageing. To be taught that, for women in particular, ageing is a one-way path to irrelevance and decay, because that's how much of the patriarchal schtick we've swallowed.)

I started where I always start, with word of mouth. I've always been a word of mouth kind of woman. If I like someone's boots on the tube I tap them on the shoulder and ask them where they got them. So I frantically fired off emails to older friends, confidently expecting them to deliver solutions straight into my lap. (Like I said, 50 going on 15). Instead, I was met with emoticon shrugs:

Me: 'Jane, when you had your menopause ...'

Jane, five years older than me and bound to be as zero tolerance on this as she is on everything else: 'I haven't. Have you? Oh my God, you poor thing. Is it shit? I heard it's shit.'

Me: 'Julia, has your menopause started ...'

Julia, two years older and one of those people who seems to know everything and everyone: 'Nope, not yet. Is it grim? I'm dreading it.'

Me, growing increasingly desperate: 'Emma ...'

Emma, four years older than me, infinitely cooler and my guiding light since I met her when we were both lowly assistants – her in PR, me in my first magazine job: 'Yep been and gone, I didn't really notice it.'

No artistic licence here, I promise. Not only were they not experiencing any symptoms – or at least none they recognised – in the main, these smart, educated, no-bull-tolerating women treated the mere possibility of menopause as if it were contagious. Like just saying the M word could bring it on. (Producer and director George, 51, told me about a choir practice where she took her jumper off and put it back on again 'about a dozen times because I was boiling. Somebody asked what was going on and I said, "Oh, menopause, hot flushes, no big deal" and people genuinely shrank back, as if I were infectious! It was a mixed group of people, around my age or slightly older. Some really powerful women. It was a funny thing. As soon as I'd said those words in that room, nothing was ever the same again and I'd been in that choir for seven years ...'). Now replace that word with another word, puberty, and imagine the same reaction. It's not even conceivable, is it? Hey, here's a seismic life change, let's just pretend it's not happening.

I did, eventually, find an ex-colleague who was not only in the midst of it, she was living her best perimenopausal life. Tania, a journalist with a special interest in 'wellness', had 'done a piece on it' (journalist-speak for 'tested my way through various bio-identical hormone treatments for free'). She was now a fully paid-up member of the Marion Gluck fan club. Gluck is arguably the biggest name in bio-identical hormones. (These differ from traditional HRT in that they're chemically identical to those produced by our bodies and derived from plant oestrogens. Let's just say that, like the rest of the HRT landscape, they're a subject of much debate. Believed by some to be the 'gold standard', others including the British Menopause Society consider them over-priced.[3] Based on Wimpole Street in central London, Gluck counts novelist Jeanette Winterson and actress Gillian Anderson among her acolytes. Winterson credits Gluck with making her feel 'at home in my body again'[4], while Anderson has said that before she met Gluck she felt like something had taken over her brain.[5] Oh, how I knew that feeling. And here was Tania, looking glossier than ever, tossing newly dyed white-blonde hair (also a perk of the job) before heading off to Bikram yoga (ditto). 'I feel better than I have for a long time,' she assured me. 'I feel like me again, but if anything a bit better.'

My instinct was to be dismissive – cynical is my MO – but it struck a chord: 'I feel like me again.' And I didn't. Right then, I'd have struggled to identify me at all.

I'm not saying there's not plenty of help to be found. If you know where to look or have the inclination to hunt for it. And there's Google. There's always Google. Try it. Go on, search 'menopause': 115 million hits and counting. There are books by the truckload and websites seem to be popping up daily. Ditto private Facebook groups if you can get an in. They can be hit and miss. Much like menopause. Anyway, my friends had drawn a blank, with one exception, and seeking help on social media (by which I mean Facebook and Instagram – can you imagine the terror of asking Twitter?!) felt like too much of a public admission that I was ageing. In the absence of anyone who 'looked like me' to ask, I muddled through, feeling lonely, depressed and very, very hot. And fat. And old. And increasingly irrelevant.

As well as raving about bio-identical hormones, Tania gave me the names of a few alternative treatments to try. Which is how I found myself in the 'mature women' section of the Women's Health aisle in Boots (it's just along from the 'fertile women' section full of ovulation predictors, pregnancy tests and the healthy pregnancy vitamins and minerals, just in case you needed reminding … It's a bit better in Holland & Barrett where it's dubbed Adult Health and lives, logically I guess, next to the Viagra equivalents). I was on the hunt for black cohosh. Given the thumbs up by countless internet forums, black cohosh is derived from the roots of a herb with Native American origins and it became popular around the same time as HRT for its supposedly oestrogen-like effects. Its best-known benefit is 'reducing night sweats' – according to one website; although according to another, those benefits are 'modest'. But it was only a tenner. Vastly cheaper than most of the other treatments on the shelves, which range from a fiver to 50 – yes, *50 quid* – for a month's supply. So I bought it. I took it, as instructed, and then I read the contraindications. This is out of character. Because I figure nine times out of ten the benefits outweigh the drawbacks (and who wants to know about the tenth?). I won't list the side effects here – you can look them up for yourself – but let's just say

25

they might conceivably be worth it, if it actually works. It didn't. Not even slightly.

Admittedly, this is a journey I was never willingly going to go on. Peppermint tea is about as woo-woo as I get, so – hands up – I was not approaching this with a Positive Mental Attitude. I took the black cohosh for a couple of weeks. The sweats kept coming. The anxiety didn't ease. The confidence kept crashing. Then I started to fixate on the side effects – usually when I was awake at 3am in the puddle of cooling sweat that wasn't meant to be there any more. Were my headaches worse? Had I gained even more weight? Was my low blood pressure even lower? Was I even dizzier? Probably not. Or if I was it probably had zero to do with black cohosh and everything to do with lying awake worrying all night, every night.

A fortnight in, I ditched the black cohosh and went through the same – increasingly expensive – process with a variety of other equally fruitless variants on a meno theme: Menopace, Menojoy, Menomood, Menocool (stick 'meno' in front of any word and it seems you give yourself a licence to print money). To be fair, any or all of them may have made a tiny difference, but it was negligible. By the time I reached the point of seriously contemplating spending £50 on a magnet to stick in my knickers (the manufacturers claim it reduces symptoms of menopause by rebalancing the autonomic nervous system and apparently Belinda Carlilse of The Go-gos – remember them, Gen Xers? – swears by it). I took it as a sign I was truly going mad enough to ditch my 'but patriarchy' principles and went in search of HRT.

There are plenty of women who swear by natural remedies – they wouldn't be produced in such quantities if there weren't – and there's certainly no shortage of rave reviews and positive feedback swarming the internet. But try as I might I couldn't find a real live one. Of the women I spoke to, most who did use supplements used them in conjunction with HRT, a healthy diet, reduced alcohol and caffeine intake and lots of exercise. Like Lisa, 52, who takes a natural supplement made of maca root. 'It helps,' she says, 'but it's not as effective as the first few packs of HRT.' Juliet, 50, takes vitamin D and magnesium; her sister tried sage, but it didn't work. Deborah, 49, tried acupuncture and Chinese medicine. But everyone I spoke to concluded that supplements were no replacement for HRT. As Nahid del Belgeonne, 52, who takes flaxseed, puts it, it's simply 'extra ammo'.

The trouble is, HRT and whether or not to take it is portrayed as a zero-sum game. You either sell your soul for oestrogen, or you go quietly but serenely into your dotage wearing art-history-teacher smocks and spending a disproportionate amount of time on hills with your dogs. Now, I want a dog as much as the next menopausal person (I have a yearning for a border terrier, as it happens – you know, the ones with little moustaches and grumpy faces) but I also want my life as I recognise it. Why should the two be mutually exclusive?

The quick answer is, they aren't. There are almost as many women who do take HRT as those who don't. (Definitive stats are on the sparse side, but the split seems to be about 40:60.) And for every one who has chosen not to take it 'because patriarchy' and because they don't want to line the pockets of the pharma-ceutical companies who are raking it in – the 'global hot flash market' was valued at $3.7 billion in 2014 and is projected to reach $5.28 billion by 2023[6] – there are two who don't take it, either because they don't consider their symptoms severe enough to warrant it, or for their own personal health reasons. Or they simply don't want to.

'I haven't taken HRT and I wouldn't because I had IVF and pumped my body so full of hormones that I'm scared to do anything else,' says Lena, 55. 'But if I'm honest, I do envy those who are on it. They seem visibly happier, younger, have more energy. Or maybe I just think they do.'

Sarah, now in her late sixties, went on HRT as soon as she experienced menopausal symptoms, largely because her mum suffered with osteoporosis. 'It had the same effect on me as going on the pill – I put on weight,' she tells me. 'So I tried another one. That was a bit better but it had a similar effect. I thought about going for a third option, but quite honestly, a full-time job, a primary school-aged child and a waste-of-space partner was enough to cope with, so I stopped taking it. A friend recommended some natural alternatives, which I took for several years. Ten years later I fell, broke my hip and was diagnosed with osteoporosis ...'

Caroline, 55, went to her doctor after 'falling into a perimenopausal hell-hole' at 50. 'I thought I was losing my mind,' she recalls. 'I was terribly anxious, suffered from dreadful night sweats, soaking wet bed every night, insomnia and rages. I cried constantly – alternately shouting and weeping. My husband and I nearly broke up. My GP whacked me on Citalopram [an antidepressant] which helped enormously.'

Why an antidepressant and not HRT? 'My GP didn't discuss HRT with me. I basically burst into her consulting room in floods. She thought I needed a helping hand. There was no mention of menopause. Citalopram saved my bacon. I came off it 18 months ago and I've felt pretty good since then.'

The antidepressant versus HRT thing is a big bone of contention. According to Paula Fry, 49, who co-founded Facebook group Feeling Flush in 2017, 'The biggest thing we hear is women being offered antidepressants instead of HRT and it makes my blood boil.' New research found that over a third of menopausal women who attend their GP are offered antidepressants before HRT.[7] 'About one in seven women will have breast cancer in their lifetime and they can't usually take HRT,' says Dr Louise Newsom[8]. 'Menopause affects everything – bones, heart, brain, sexual identity. We need to focus more on the health risks for older women of not being on HRT and stop repeating the canard about HRT being dangerous.'

Others have similar personal health reasons for eschewing HRT, many of which are related to cancer – their own or that of close family members. Writer Stella Duffy, 56, first had breast cancer and subsequent early menopause 20 years ago. It recurred ten years later. 'If people want to take HRT, go for it,' she says. 'But I wouldn't risk it – I don't have hormonal cancer so I *could* take it, but personally I feel high risk, so I'm not chancing it. Also, now my symptoms are much more manageable so it's not like I'm "WTF can I do?" It might be different if that were the case ... Having been through what I've been through I love the places where my body is doing stuff of itself rather than being forced into it through drugs ... I have a desire to be the age I am and that is from not being dead at 36. I like being 56. I think it's fucking amazing that I'm 56 and I'm still here. So if I hurt, if I have a hot flush, I want to be me in my body, not two separate things.'

Her partner, writer Shelley Silas, 61, has a different approach. For most of her perimenopause, she was a vocal HRT refusenik. But two weeks before we spoke, something changed. 'For ages I would have a go at women for taking HRT,' she admits, 'I once said to a friend on Twitter, "How *can* you take it? What's wrong with you?" But now, oh my God, I get it. I get your body being pushed to a limit where you're just not able to function and it prevents you doing things; you worry about going out and just dripping sweat. I got quite desperate. I felt like one more hot flush and I would kill someone. That's how bad it was. I just wanted to feel normal, human.

'I couldn't cope,' she continues. 'I couldn't cope with my mum [Shelley's sister died nine years ago, leaving her to look after her mum, who's 92, with the help of a carer; a common situation for women in mid-life] and work and life and, on top of all that, every half an hour feeling like I was melting. I'd fought against it for so long because of the risks I thought it involved. But it got to the point where it was actually making me mad, so I just went to the GP. I take back everything I ever said and all my harsh judgements. I used to be quite vitriolic telling people it wouldn't make them younger inside, but I see now that HRT is not about wanting to be younger, it's about feeling better about yourself. It's an internal thing not a vanity thing. I thought I could deal with it and I couldn't. That's nothing to be embarrassed about.'

Desperation is a common thread among many women who opt for HRT, but it's not always that dramatic. For journalist Kate Spicer, 50, who has just started taking HRT, it wasn't a question of if but when. 'Gen X have done a lot of drugs – some more than others,' she says with a shrug. 'But honestly if I can spend the first 30 years of my adult life sniffing coke and taking pills, I can spend the next 30 taking hormones!'

Joanna Davies, 52, founder of Black White Denim boutique in Cheshire, experienced a massive confidence crisis and depression that affected her ability to manage her staff and bring up her family. To her, HRT was a 'no-brainer'. 'I wanted to be in control of my emotions, not at the mercy of my hormones,' she says matter-of-factly. 'I see it as taking a supplement, just as I would a vitamin or probiotic. I am low in oestrogen so I take it via a gel. I'm low in vitamin C so I take it in a tablet. To me it's exactly the same principle and I had no qualms about it.'

But many who eventually take HRT sound like I felt: exhausted, unable to cope, desperate to 'just feel like a human again'. Time and again I've heard the same things: 'I was sick of wading through treacle just to get through the day.' 'It was making me crazy.' 'I tried to navigate my way through this on my own but it got to the point where I couldn't.' 'I had brain fog, I couldn't think clearly, which spiralled into days where I couldn't even begin to function.' 'It got to the stage where menopause was seriously affecting my quality of life. I couldn't cope with everyday stresses and felt like I was living in a dark cloud.' 'I didn't know who I was any more.'

According to suicide figures produced by The Samaritans in 2018, the age group for women with the highest suicide rate per 100,000 in the UK is 50–54. The average age of menopause is 51 ... I don't think that's a coincidence. As Shelley said, 'it's an internal thing not a vanity thing'. It's about taking back control of your life, not looking younger. For those women and the millions like them, the decision whether or not to take HRT is a mental health issue.

I can say that now, with the absolute clarity afforded me by Femoston Conti 1/5mg, but at the time, it was a big deal for me, 'because patriarchy'. I felt I *shouldn't* take HRT, that it was fundamentally wrong, that I would be letting down not just myself but ALL WOMEN, siding with the male medical establishment and boosting the coffers of the already loaded and morally dubious pharmaceutical industry into the bargain. I was nervous of being judged and found wanting. I've always cared too much what other people think. I'm not alone in that. It's taken me until now to see it as the debilitating and pointless waste of effort it really is. But, yes, I am the idiot who did not seek the medication that would immeasurably improve my life just in case an acquaintance, or a young woman at work, or someone's mum, or some random shouty person on the internet, disapproved. I know. So much for giving zero fucks. (Those came, but they took a while longer to arrive.)

Like everything to do with women's health, HRT is public property, subject to judgement and endless scare stories. But then if you've grown up female, you'll be used to that by now. Making the decision to take oestrogen (if you do it publicly – and why should we have to hide it?) puts you on the sharp edge of public opinion. As Marina Benjamin so succinctly put it in her book *The Middlepause*, 'any decision to take oestrogen is political'. It shouldn't be. But it is. Take it, don't take it. Take bio-identicals, take body-identicals (which have the same molecular structure as the hormones in your body). Take oestrogen, take progestogen, take it combined, add testosterone. Take a pill, use a cream, wear a patch. (That invariably spends more time stuck to your knickers than your leg ...) And that's before you get into the potential risks. (Depending on which bit of research you believe.) It's a minefield.

I read books that HRT-shamed me and made me feel like a man-pleasing tool of the patriarchy who had internalised the male gaze to such an extent that I was prepared to medicalise a natural state of being. I read books that were so evangelically in HRT's favour that I suspected they might have been taking a cut, so it goes both ways. But the 'cool girls' didn't approve and I have always wanted to be a cool girl so for a while I let myself be shamed. Plus, there was a part of me who wanted to be 'that woman', the elegant coper, the one who swanned through meno-pause and out the other side with barely a symptom and hardly a (silver) hair out of place, but I couldn't see her for the brain fog. If I had been able to, I'd probably have discovered that she took HRT, too.

And that, to me, is the clincher. Because while we still know woefully little about menopause, as we enter this phase of our lives we have even less agency over our own bodies (and, equally importantly, our minds) than ever. Whether or not you're opposed to HRT, a significant minority of GPs are still reluctant to prescribe it. Bestselling author Marian Keyes, 56, summed it up: 'My GP wants to stop my HRT because of breast cancer worries. (I've no history of it.) I would prefer the risk of breast cancer than to go mad again, but I'm not given that agency over my own body.' Speaking personally, I was losing it big time and I wanted it back. I'm entitled to make that decision. Me. Not a doctor. Not my partner. Not some berk on the internet. As usual, we are shooting ourselves in the foot (knees, even), pitting women against women – the HRT-takers versus the tough-it-outers, the natural versus the chemical, the bio-identical versus the body-identicals, the women's agency versus the tool of the patriarchy – when we'd be better off fighting for one thing: each individual woman's right to make her own informed decision, regardless of income, postcode and GP. Give us the facts, let us make up our own minds.

Kate Spicer agrees. 'That thing of it being an empowering brilliant time of life is true, but it's spoiled by the hormonal shit that stops you enjoying the boost in power. I don't want to suffer. I've suffered enough. The hormones are important to me and I object to being made to feel like I'm doing something wrong.'

That was the point I'd reached when I hurled my soggy, fog-addled self on my gynaecologist's mercy. I'd made my peace with my feminist credentials. I didn't feel good about the whole patriarchy thing but what use was I to society – patriarchal or otherwise – if I couldn't even string a sentence together half the time? If a friend had come to me in exactly the same position and asked my advice, I'd have said the same, without hesitation. (And shortly after I started taking HRT, one did.) It was that, combined with my complete inability to function as a human being, that made me decide HRT was worth a try for me.

As I've said before, I was lucky. Claire knew my gynaecological history inside out. She knew it was chequered and she had to go easy on the progestogen. And we didn't get it right first time. That would have been too easy. I tried an oestrogen cream and two-weekly progestogen pill – the progestogen didn't suit me. I tried bio-identical – they did F-all. And finally I tried a compound pill (the Femoston Conti 1/5mg I mentioned earlier). Within days of taking it, the brain fog lifted, the night sweats and the day storms eased up and with them the 3am, 5am, 9am anxiety attacks. I looked and felt better because I was no longer an overheated insomniac with a permanent headache, not because of some miracle. Yes, I was still inclined to be depressed and lacking in confidence, but in a way I recognised. It's HRT not a personality transformer. To quote Marion Gluck: 'Self-esteem and contentment can't be compounded in a cream to be applied twice daily.' I wish.

Right now, I still take HRT. And I feel pretty good. Most of the time. It's three years since I've had a period (give or take, I'm not counting). I don't miss them. Not even slightly. I have annual check-ups and I can't envisage stopping HRT any time soon. It's part of my life. But maybe I will. Who knows? Maybe, like my friend Clare, I'll just forget to pack my pills when I go on holiday one time and realise, when I haven't taken them for a week or two, that I don't need them any more. That I'm the same without them as I am with. Post-menopausal me. Free.

'Hormonal treatment is not a miracle cure for misogyny. Society does not value older women and, often, older women do not value themselves.'

Dr Marion Gluck

2

THE EXPIRY DATE

Redefining the point of you when society has
decided you no longer have one. AKA why women
over 50 are 'past it' but men are in their prime

My second brush with mortality was sitting in my beloved blue
Mini facing the wrong way, half on, half off a busy road somewhere in Shropshire as traffic streamed past in both directions. I
was 20. I was driving my housemates from university in
Birmingham to a friend's 21st birthday party near Shrewsbury. In
that moment, I came very close to killing myself and my three
closest friends. Seconds earlier we had been facing forward, travelling at probably 50, maybe 60, miles an hour. We were definitely
talking – as we did all the time, all at the same time, all over each
other. Something was playing, probably The Cure or the Cocteau
Twins. It's a cliché to say it happened in a split second, but it felt
that way. A Volvo twice our size pulled out from behind and accel-
erated to overtake. As the Volvo loomed in my wing mirror, an
articulated lorry appeared from nowhere, bearing down in front.
There wasn't time for the Volvo to get past. There wasn't room for
him to pull in front if he did. So I did what every driving instructor
in the land would tell you not to do: I braked to let him in,
skidded and lost control of the car. I remember spinning the steer-
ing wheel, probably in the wrong direction. I remember the Mini

careering into the path of the oncoming lorry and out again, back into the path of the car behind. Then we were hanging off the hard shoulder, facing backwards, both lorry and Volvo gone. The car behind us stopped and the driver ran back to see if we were all right and offered to call the police. We mumbled that we were fine. Not sure why. Concussion perhaps. Or, more likely, because we were four very young women and who was going to listen to us anyway? The owner of a nearby farmhouse took us in and made us tea, helped me check the car over and let us use his phone to call the friend whose party we were on our way to. (No mobile phones, it was that long ago.)

Miraculously neither the car nor two of my friends were injured. Not so much as a burst tyre. The following day we discovered my friend Jill who'd been sitting behind me had a fractured shoulder. Later I found I had fractured my pelvis.

I started with my second near-death experience because it's the easiest to recount. The least painful. If I'm going to be honest with myself, the first time I truly feared for my life was before that. I was locked in a bathroom. Not for the first time. Although this time I had at least locked myself in there. The bathroom was in a small studio – secluded, covetable, private – in the gardens of a three-star hotel, somewhere in the Mediterranean. (One of those last-minute pay-five-hundred-quid-for-a-fortnight go-where-we-send-you holidays.) I was almost two thousand miles from home. I was scared. I was sober. And I was fully aware that in this bath-room, in this micro-villa with no adjoining rooms, no rooms above or below, no one could hear me scream. Well, one person could. He was the reason I had locked myself in the bathroom in the first place. He, I can only assume, got a kick out of my terror. It wasn't the first time. But I'm going to spoil the suspense right now by telling you it *was* the last. He (my boyfriend of quite some time) ranted, railed and raged outside, while I sat on the lid of the toilet shivering in fear and wondering how the hell I was going to get out of here. Then he stopped. And instead of the torrent of abuse there was only silence. The silence was worse. I had trapped myself in a tiled six-by-four box, with no windows and no way out other than the door I'd just locked, on the other side of which awaited ice-cold fury. Lips so tight and thin they'd vanished. Grey eyes hard as stone. ('What was the worst thing that could happen?' a therapist asked me more than 30 years later. I pretended to think about it, though I was certain of the answer. He'd hurt me before. But right then, in that room, far from anywhere, I thought he might do worse.) I could have stayed in that sterile en suite all night. Hoping like hell that by morning he would have crashed out, his fury blown over. But I didn't. I was done. I undid the lock and opened the door. He was sat on the bed, waiting for me. He did his worst. It hurt, a lot, but it wasn't as bad as it could have been. I'm here now, aren't I? The next morning, I got up, went to the hotel reception and insisted we change rooms. The noisiest, most public available, with rooms on all sides and ideally a balcony that was overlooked, bin lorry that came past at 4am if it came to it. He didn't try to stop me. Maybe he didn't recognise me – with the benefit of hindsight, I'm not sure I recognised myself. Maybe this new me scared him. Who knows? I wasn't afraid of him any more. For the rest of the holiday, he didn't harm me and when we got home, I dumped him. I didn't die, but that night I knew how it felt to believe you might.

And then there was the cancer scare in my mid-thirties. I'm not going to make a meal of that. It was just that, a scare. An unexplained lump at the base of my neck that, after endless tests and much blank-faced shaking of medical heads, turned out to be a floating rib. It floats there still. It was briefly frightening and it made me feel mortal, but even just thinking about it now I feel fortunate, because in the intervening 20 years I have had so many friends who weren't. Friends in remission, friends who've relapsed, friends who've died. Family, friends, incredible women much admired from afar. Three bright brilliant women, shining lights, all snuffed out by cancer as I wrote this book. Just three of the many, many women around my age who don't get to be here to moan about the menopause and getting a bit older, a bit flabbier, a bit more forgetful.

All my brushes with mortality were just ... normal. The type of stories most of us have tucked away in our memory bank by the time we reach our life's mid-way point. Cancer scares (or not), car crashes, terrifying walks home with our keys wedged between our knuckles, relationships that can best be described as a learning experience. Which, just in case you were wondering where the hell I was going with this, does bring me back to the menopause, because the onset of menopause was a brush with mortality I hadn't reckoned with. I'm not saying it made me fear for my life, so much as for my life as I had known it. For a while the 'socially useful' self I had spent so long shaping wavered. In her place, a woman who at best could be described as a mirage. In an attempt to sum up how this felt I turned to the dictionary and discovered a word that had truthfully never occurred to me before: *moribund*. Broadly, it means 'no more use for' or 'being in a state of obsolescence'. Or even more cheerfully 'about to come to an end'. Like shipyards and telephone tables and TV listings magazines. Redundant. Over. History. You know when you hear people describe you as 'the former xxx' or 'she used to be xxx'? It's that, applied to your entire life. It's not so much coming face-to-face with your imminent demise, as being served with evidence that like the eggs you no longer have, your expiry date has come, your usefulness to society, such as it was, has been outlived.

Moribund. That was how I felt.

While I'm inclined to be glass-half-empty, I'm neither defeatist nor a giver-upper. I've been thriving on proving people wrong ever since a journalism lecturer at an interview for college told me I didn't have what it takes to make it in magazines. So this sense of utter pointlessness floors me. Having quit my job to work on a start-up with a friend only a few months earlier, I flounder. (With the benefit of hindsight, the job-quitting was likely the start of it ... I honestly don't regret it, but I can't pretend it wasn't a borderline insane, not to mention selfish, thing to do.) Suddenly I was stuck in a spiral of self-doubt of my own making: what if I'm no good at anything any more? What if no one wants me? What if I am, as I'm starting to fear, past my sell-by date?

This hollowness is partly internal. A combined product of my always over-active inner critic ('making me feel not good enough since 1966') and the anxiety/brain fog/sleeplessness that took up residence along with perimenopause. As George, 51, put it, 'I just thought I was a piece of crap!' But let's be honest, it's not just that is it? Because in order to feel useless you have to have a pretty clear idea of what use*ful* means and that, it will not surprise you, depends very much on who wrote the definition of useful. A clue: not you, nor anyone who looks like you. As American writer Darcey Steinke puts it in her brilliant menopause memoir-come-anthropological study, *Flash Count Diary*, 'Instead of new obsessions and responsibilities I feel a nothingness, a negation. It's a void created in part by an oversexed patriarchal culture that has little room for older women. The message, never stated directly but manifesting in myriad ways, is an overwhelmingly nihilistic one. Your usefulness is over. Please step to the sidelines.'

In short, get out of the way old woman/hag/crone (pick your derogatory epithet of choice) and let the important people get on with their busy-work: the young men, the middle-aged men, the mature and worldly men (natch) and the young women. (And, yes, you can almost definitely preface all of those with white and straight and (upper) middle class and able-bodied.) Because they are 'useful'. Women who aren't even fertile any more? Whose vaginas are shrunken, wombs shrivelled and ovaries empty? Not so much.

There's a quote that's stuck with me ever since I first saw it. It so resonated that I instantly wrote it down in my Notes app on my phone and it lives there still: 'A woman is ... set up as a pregnancy machine.' It's by Dr Jane Dickson, Consultant in Sexual and Reproductive Health Care at the Royal College of Obstetrics and Gynaecology, and it's taken from an interview she did with journalist Eleanor Morgan for her book *Hormonal*. It's also vastly less offensive than the comment New York internist Dr Erika Schwartz made to journalist Christa D'Souza when she was researching her book *The Hot Topic*: 'Once you lose your hormones, you are nothing more than roadkill.' Youch.

Then, shortly after, came *that Fleabag* episode. No, not the 'kneel' one, the one with Kristin Scott Thomas. The one where her character, Belinda, somewhere in her mid-late fifties, wit as bone-dry as her martinis, cheekbones like wing mirrors, jaded as hell, says this: 'The menopause comes, and it is the most wonderful fucking thing in the world. Yes, your entire pelvic floor crumbles and you get fucking hot and no one cares, and then ... you're free. No longer a slave, no longer a machine, with parts. You're just a person ... It's horrendous. But then it's magnificent.'

It's my phone's screen saver, it's on the wall above my desk, it's the preface to this book. I could quote it in my sleep. And there's a reason for that. I had never before seen anyone talk about meno-pause in a mainstream drama or comedy in a way that wasn't self-mocking, self-loathing or both. Menopausal women were either overheated rage buckets without a waist or glossy and pneumatic with faces like clingfilm, still as lithe as when they were 25 and boy did they work at it. These women would die – probably quite literally – before they'd let the M-word pass their lips. But here was a woman who was in between. She was funny, she was smart, she didn't give a flying fuck – and she was post-menopau-sal. Oh, and she was still hot. Fleabag fancied her. *I* fancied her. It was like a lightbulb going on. A whole string of lightbulbs. But also. ALSO. It plugged straight into what Dickson said. If society sees you as primarily useful for one thing and one thing only – begetting, having, bringing up babies – what comes next? It's not *quite* as overt as that, of course. As Steinke says in *Flash Count*

Diary, it's never stated directly, but when it came for me, I couldn't help feeling very conscious that a certain tranche of the population (and not all of it male) didn't know what to do with me any more than I did. They would have been happier if they could have given me my regulation menopause smock and dog of choice, and sent me packing along with my social P45. Instead, some of them did the second-best thing and pretended I was no longer there.

I have never had children, and it has never occurred to me to value myself by the fecundity of my eggs. I would have been on a hiding to nothing if I had. As a partner, a lover, a journalist, an editor, a friend, a mentor, a surrogate adult, yes, all of those contributed to what millennial actress and activist Jameela Jamil calls my 'weight'. But eggs? No. I wasn't oblivious to the patriarchy. I'm not stupid. Like most other women of my age and class – and to a lesser or greater degree women of all ages, classes and races – I've been contorting myself into ever more uncomfortable shapes to accommodate society's expectations of girls like me, since I was old enough to walk. From the moment I had a little brother I knew that the differences in the way we were treated, the expectations on us, particularly in the domestic sphere, were down to more than the fact that I was the eldest.

I knew, long before I went to comprehensive school, that girls who were pretty got a pass and that they had a window of opportunity to capitalise on that. And capitalise on it was what they were expected to do, by grabbing the most conventionally handsome, fittest (in both senses) boy they could find and nailing him down sharpish. (Some methods were more frowned upon than others, but needs must.) Where I come from, that was the pinnacle of achievement: meeting a nice boy (probably good at sport) who got a good job, buying a nice house and producing a family, and living Happily Ever After. I know it sounds like the 1950s, but it's the story that's been laid out for women for centuries and it hasn't changed as much as we'd like to think in the last 50-odd years. Anyway, I was ginger, freckly, dumpy, a bomb at pretty much all sports, singing voice like two foxes mating and absolutely zero sense of rhythm. I've also been cursed with resting bitch face from the moment I came out of the womb upside down (I'm not blaming the forceps, it's just my face). I figured out pretty early that I was going to have to find another way to earn society's approval.

And then came periods and from the minute the first girl in my class 'started' the world's plan for us all became clear. Angie was ten. Ten. And yet suddenly she was a sexual being, or was starting to be perceived as such. News of her new 'grown up' state went viral in the playground. The boys immediately treated her differently, as if her menstruation had flicked some switch in them, too. The teachers – male and female – started, imperceptibly at first, keeping her at arm's length. She was no longer a little girl and as such could not be treated like one. She was ten FFS. And the other girls? We flocked to her – or we fled. Awe and longing or sheer unadulterated terror. We wanted to be her, but at the same time she terrified us. The power of her. It was too much for ten-year-old me. God knows how it felt being her. She was young, she was beautiful, she was fertile. (Yes, she was ten. In some cultures and historical eras she'd have been married.) Her place in the world was assigned, and soon, as ten became eleven and primary school became comprehensive and eleven became twelve became thirteen, we were all initiated into this new world of womanhood – a world that came, back then, with unexpected pain, more blood than we'd been led to believe, and a creepy nun called Sister Marian courtesy of Procter & Gamble. Our roles were allotted: the sexy one, the pretty one, the sporty one and, if you were very unlucky, the swotty one. But we all knew the truth: the sexy, pretty ones were the most sought after, the ones at the top of the girl tree.

I hadn't heard the phrase 'male gaze' before I went to university but I had already internalised it. I knew it had looked me over once or twice, and found me wanting. And the more I dismissed it, the more I subconsciously wanted to please it. Secretly I wanted a boyfriend more than I cared to admit – mainly because everyone else had one. Ditto losing my virginity. But at the same time I rejected it as hard and fast as I could. It was the mid-80s, whatever wave of feminism that was, we were all Greenham Common and CND, Reclaim the Night marches and a reading list that came solely from a relatively new publisher called Virago that only published books by women. Such a thing was unheard of! Margaret Atwood and Angela Carter were my gods, the music of the Cocteau Twins' Liz Fraser became the soundtrack to my first year. I loved Sinead O'Connor and Nico and didn't really understand the damage society was inflicting on them. I became a goth and dyed my hair black, dressed exclusively in clothes from Birmingham's Digbeth market (behind the bus station) and lived 24/7 in Dr Martens. (Some things never change.) If society wouldn't love me, well, I wouldn't love it. But it was all just armour. Deep inside, it was just an act. If I'd been shown some love, I would have contorted myself into all kinds of shapes to fit its expectations of me, which is how I ended up locked in the bathroom earlier in this chapter.

When I started out in journalism – writing 'true life stories' for weekly magazines *Chat* and then *Take A Break* before moving to monthly glossies – the world was a different place. We'd had three waves of feminism and things were undeniably changing, but it still wasn't possible, for instance, in the eyes of the English law for a man to rape his wife (that didn't change until 1991). Men still routinely got away with killing their wives on the grounds they were driven to it, poor lambs, by those annoying, nagging, cuckolding women. Needless to say, women in the same situation weren't cut the same sort of slack. In the early 90s, I and the outspoken young women I worked with on *Chat* spent as many pages as we could get away with championing women's issues, disguised as real-life stories. Because, you know, women's stories *are* real-life stories. Stories like those of Kiranjit Ahluwalia,

Sara Thornton and Emma Humphreys, three women who were serving life for murdering their abusive husbands. It wasn't technically what we were there for but our boss Terry (a warm, compassionate woman in her late forties, a hardworking single mum of two teenagers with an eye for talent and a wry sense of humour) gave us as much rope as she reasonably could without jeopardising her job, and we took it willingly. And then some. I owe her more than I can say – and her influence on me and my subsequent management style was enormous, not that I ever managed to be as fun or as generous a boss as she. But it's only now, as I write this, that I realise that, when I'd moved on to the next job, eyes on the prize, it was not long before she went on her way too; the way of all female editors her age.

The concept of invisibility simply hadn't occurred to me then. I had big ginger hair that, like it or not, had always made me visible and I had learnt to match that with a big mouth. I did know about being 'past it'. (*It* being some sort of unspoken but indelible expiry date. You might not be able to see it with the naked eye, but it was there all the same. Like invisible ink, you just needed to know where and how to look. Although this ink seemed to be curiously chromosome specific. That notion was so ingrained that, when I was made editor of *Company* magazine, my third editorship, at just 32, I wondered aloud to a media journalist whether I should be lying about my age. Thirty-two. I ask you.)

I, like other young journalists fast tracking it to editorship, hell bent on getting to the top regardless, paid little attention to the women – because it was almost always women – going the other way. That their apparent waning relevance had more to do with their age and their faces and their bodies no longer fitting – their perceived biddability waning with their increasing years – than their talent and ability to do their jobs didn't occur to me. Why would it? It didn't apply to me. (One (male) boss I had – a happy reactionary – once looked around the table at an awards ceremony and announced proudly, 'Well you can say one thing for [this company]. We don't employ mingers.' The only person much above 40 and male was him. Yes, I was shocked. And disgusted. But it was far from the first time I'd heard something of that nature and I did not stop working for him.) But I did clock that it didn't seem to apply to their male peers and I filed it away to be dissected at a later date. I know now, of course, that those women were probably also far more expensive than me, having earned their way to substantial six-figure salaries. By replacing an experienced, well-connected woman with a younger, 'more relevant' face you could get two for the price of one. So it wasn't just ageism and sexism, although it was definitely those, but an economic decision, too. One that could equally have applied to their male peers. But strangely never did. At the time, though, I simply didn't see. I didn't want to.

What I did see as I climbed the ladder and reached that much-coveted glass box on the fourth floor – still wearing my Converse; a micro rebellion, since I had the regulation pile of over-priced unwalkable Jimmy Choos and Louboutins under my desk – was that the more senior you became the more homogenous the faces. They fell into two camps: women predominantly under 40 and men. And, yes, at that time, all white. Especially the women. Mostly on the thin side. Especially the women. Gotta fit in those sample sizes ... And mostly, unlike me, middle or upper middle class. They were undoubtedly not all straight (but outside the confines of fashion, they still felt obliged to play those cards extremely close to their chest). By the time they reached 50, the women were all gone. Nowhere to be seen. Now I know why.

Which brings me back to babies. From the age of 26, when I got married, until my early 40s, I was asked one of the following questions at least once a week: did I have children? Was I going to have children? When was I going to have children? Did I want children? If not, why not? Was I not able to have children? And later, did I regret not having children? By friends, family, colleagues, bosses (yes, I know it's illegal, it was then, too) and even total strangers. Aside from the fact it was none of their bloody business, show me any man ever who has been asked these questions even once, let alone once a week.

Now I am no longer theoretically childbearing and have outlived my so-called reproductive usefulness, the questions have – finally, blissfully – stopped, but with them so has the sense of purpose society deigns to bestow on me. Or should that be inflict? As my last egg trickled away, society lost the plot – or, rather, it ran out of plot. Its storyline is limited where women are concerned: husband, babies, house, happy ever after. That's it? For 50+ per cent of the population? Poet and essayist Katha Pollitt puts it best when she says, 'This story not only fails to fill a lifetime, it puts the plotline in the hands of others.' Those others being men. I suppose, in its defence, it's not so long ago that we were expected to have a baby or five, in quick succession, then die and be replaced by a younger model. A lifetime was 40. Or 50, tops. But now, in 2020, when we're only halfway through our lives and expecting, quite reasonably, to live, laugh, work and create – just *be* – well into the next half, if we're lucky, that plot's just not good enough.

'I know so many amazing 50+ women who have had a crisis of confidence, as I did, just not really knowing where I belonged,' says Lena, 55, a writer with two sons, both now in their twenties. 'And it wasn't bloody empty nest syndrome – which is what everyone always assumes, which in itself pisses me off. When did you last hear anyone say a man was suffering from empty nest syndrome? It makes me seethe.'

Lena is one of many women who've told me they feel their mid-life status is regarded as a joke, both by peers and younger women. 'I'm about to be a grandmother,' she continues. 'Everyone comments on it and several people have started calling me "Granny", but few people have laughed at the idea of my husband being Granddad. In fact, even though he's only a year younger than me, nobody ever mentions his age at all.

'It's the fact the world looks at us differently once we age and so we look at ourselves differently sometimes, too.' (This is so, so true; when I asked Kate Spicer if she'd ever been age-shamed, her frank response was: 'The only person who age-shames me is me.') Back to Lena: 'Truthfully I have never been worried about my age or lied about it, and have always felt that getting older is a privilege many don't have – but I just hate the way it's a constant joke, people assume you don't want to be "old" if you're a woman. I'm more aware than ever how different life is for men when they get older. They're "silver foxes". What are we? Little grey-haired old ladies? This misogyny is so deeply ingrained.'

It is. But maybe the time has come for us to take control; to turn the gaze around and stop internalising it. Yes, my eggs have expired. No doubt about it. They're long gone. But the rest of me is still here and firing on more cylinders than ever. Not so much storyless, as story-free. In fact, I feel a new plotline coming on.

'The freedom that comes from no longer being fertile is huge.'

Cynthia Nixon

3

THE LAST EGG

Coping with the end of fertility even if
you were never fertile anyway

I am sitting in a puddle in the ladies' loos. The puddle is coming
from me. My head, my neck, my armpits, my crotch, the backs of
my knees. My ankles. My elbows. Even my belly is sweating. My
whole body is running with it. I am on fire. My clothes are
drenched. I have meetings all day and I don't know what to do.

On the other side of the paper-thin divider I can hear someone
crying in the next loo. Despite the fact there are at least a dozen
companies in this office building, four on this floor alone, I'm
pretty sure I know who it is. And I think I know why she is
crying. She is TTC (trying to conceive, I'm reliably informed) and
having IVF and she cries almost all the time. She thinks I don't
know, but I've known lots of people who've had a lot of IVF and
every single one of them has cried almost all the time. Before,
because they couldn't conceive, the tumultuous agony of the
unwanted blood month in, month out; during, because of the
endless hormone injections that pick up their emotions and hurl
them rag-doll-like at the wall when they're least expecting it (and,
yes, give them a fake, short-lived menopause ...); and after, when
they either don't conceive or, worse, do conceive but miscarry.
Again. And again. And again.

Right now, as I listen to her choking sobs, I want to add my pain to hers. The best part of 15 years divides us, but we have far more in common than she realises. I, too, cannot conceive. And, now, I never will. No amount of IVF will make the slightest difference, because I am all out of eggs.

All. Out. Of. Eggs.

Even now those four words leave me feeling hollowed out. An emptiness I have never experienced and never expected to. The emptiness of the never-will-be mother. Leaving aside, for the moment, the fact that for most of my adult life I never particularly wanted to be.

But it's only now the eggs have gone that the consequences have fully sunk in. I was about 40 when Claire, the gynaecologist you met in Chapter 1, told me my eggs were running out. After a lifetime of gynaecological mayhem, I'd been pointed in her direction by Brigid, the health editor of *Red* magazine, where I was then editor. Claire never once made me feel like the total liability/mad woman that had become a feature of my futile appointments with various GPs. (BTW I'm not dissing the NHS. Far from it. It's a lifesaver. Those people are living saints. But when it comes to GPs and my vagina, it has been less than great.) Ironically, Claire's specialism is IVF and the corridor outside her consulting room is plastered with pictures of her success stories: ecstatic mothers, fathers and babies beaming with love and joy. I guess it follows that sorting out the various gynaecological problems that impede conception would be part of Claire's skill set. Polyps, fibroids, menorrhagia, dysmenorrhea, adenomyosis, you name it I had it, and Claire, over the previous few years, had dealt with it. At this point, my periods still involved Hammer Horror levels of blood (think a super plus tampon and a pad the size of a nappy and if I was lucky that would last me the hour and fifteen minutes it took to get to work), but compared to a couple of years earlier they were positively light.

It was while I was lying on a plastic examination couch, naked from the waist down, blanket over my thighs to preserve my non-existent modesty, with an ultrasound wand thrust inside my vagina, that she said it.

'See,' she said, turning to her computer and using the mouse to draw a fluorescent-green rhombus around a fuzzy area of dark grey pixels on the screen that hung above my feet.

'Uh-huh.' I nodded, studiously non-committal. I couldn't see, but by this point I'd had enough ultrasound scans to have become practised at pretending I knew exactly what she was talking about.

'I don't think we need to do a partial hysterectomy, after all,' she said triumphantly.

Hysterectomy? Where did that come from?

'That's great, but ... why?' I ventured, hoping I sounded sufficiently grateful.

'You're almost out of eggs,' she said, as if she were looking in a fridge and not my ovaries. Not unkindly, but with the pragmatism of a woman whose day is full of wombs and there's nothing particularly special about this one. No more eggs = no more buckets of blood. Every cloud etc. 'You'll probably go into peri-menopause soon anyway, so there's no point putting you through an operation for the sake of a matter of months. A year at most.'

I nodded. Did more non-committal grunting, put my knickers back on and went to work.

Over the years I had developed quite the talent for putting out of my mind things I really didn't want in it, so that's what I did with that piece of information. I went back to work, carried on bleeding and swiftly forgot about it. As it turned out, I didn't go into perimenopause within the year as she predicted. Instead I bled, had more polyps removed, bled less, had more fibroids removed, bled even less, and then, slowly, my periods did dribble to a halt. Then I bled again and had a very painful D&C, minus any anaesthetic, to scrape out the thickening walls of my uterus.

('Shall we just get it over with?' 'Yes!' said my obedient, traitor-ous, stupid mouth. 'No fucking way!' shrieked my whole being. Afterwards I threw up.) Then the bleeding stopped, started again, and then stopped for what turned out to be the last time. In total this probably took around three years. I didn't pay much atten-tion, I just got on with life. I am – or was – master of the art of being so busy you don't have to think about it. Any of it.

And now, here I was. Sat in the ladies, working out how to put my game face on, all the while with my soggy knickers clinging to my bum, listening to another woman's sobs echo around the cubicle and realising that the damp that had my hair slicked to my neck and that was drenching the front of my shirt was not just sweat. I was crying, silently, alongside her.

For the babies I would never have. For the mother I would never be.

If this sounds self-indulgent, I guess it is. A bit. I'd never really been broody. The tick of the biological clock that so haunts some women, reaching a crescendo that's impossible to ignore, had only occasionally sounded in my head. My career had always come first – it's a cliché to say my jobs were my babies, but they were; first magazines, then books and then The Pool. I was proud of the things I and my teams created, proud of the difference we tried to make, proud of what I saw as my ability to spot talent: the fierce, quick-witted young women I took on, trained and sent on their way as grown writers and journalists. All of them a part of me in their way. Even if society doesn't see it that way. My fertility had always been reluctant at best. In both directions: yes, I was reluctant, but so was it. There were few scares in my 30-odd so-called fertile years after the one, at university. I was an absolute mess, emotionally, psychologically, physically, every-thing-lly. My weight was below seven stone, my mental health was hanging by a thread. I was terrified and trapped. I didn't think twice. All I really remember was the terror and then the relief. I got up, I got better (sort of), I graduated.

It was the mid-80s, the age of women Having It All, the heyday of Helen Gurley Brown's *Cosmopolitan*. Then *Elle* launched, then *Marie Claire*. All aimed at intelligent young women on a mission to do things and go places. The advent of 'the career woman'. Women's magazines fat with glossy ads abounded with images of smart working women, hair neat, clothes immaculate, face perfectly made up with a briefcase under one arm and a baby under the other as they made decisions that changed the world and still got home in time for supper. Oh, how we laughed. Or we would have done, if any of us had had the energy.

I never really bought the whole Having It All thing. Don't get me wrong, I think it's a wonderful aspiration and I applaud anyone who can pull it off. I know several women who appear to have done just that – from the outside, at least: the sparkling high-paying career, the gorgeous house, the tumble of kids and dogs, the happy-enough marriage, the partner who pulls their weight. I'm sure it's not as easy as their Instagrams make it look. I'm just grateful to have some of it. I always was. The 'some of it' was a career and, if I was lucky, a person who loved me enough to put up with me. I decided early on that if something had to give – and I believed in my heart that it did – the world could live without a mini-me in it.

I thought I was OK with that. Actually, scrap that, I *am* OK with it. The occasional waves of sadness during perimenopause have passed. I have children in my life. In my mid-twenties I lucked in to a stepson I adore, and now, thanks to him, have a god-daughter/step-granddaughter – and though my partner and I never tried *not* to get pregnant, I also never conceived. At the point my friends were embarking on round after round of relationship- and bank-balance-annihilating IVF, we decided not to put ourselves through it. If I got pregnant, well, great. And if I didn't, well, we'd live with that, too. What would be, would be.

But in that cubicle, after years of secret relief when the tell-tale cramp began and blood appeared in my knickers, I was filled with a profound sense of loss. And had been, I realised then, for months. In truth, there were days when I couldn't distinguish it from the depression, anxiety and general lack of confidence that accompanied the drop in oestrogen, but it was there nonetheless. I had never experienced the baby hunger some of my friends who are mothers describe. (You know, when somebody posts a picture of a pudgy-kneed just-past-newborn on Facebook and your time-line fills with exploding ovaries?) But lately I had felt my eyes fill with tears as a woman breastfed a newborn baby next to me in a coffee shop. I'd suppressed the urge to reach out and stroke the hair of a passing toddler – only realising it was creepy just in time. I'd made goo-goo faces at babies peering at me over a parental shoulder. I had lain awake at 3am and wondered, futilely, what a mini-us might have looked like. All of this in my mid-late forties. Before? Not so much.

It was only as I sat there, listening to another woman's very real grief as the hormones lashed at her defences, that the reality of my situation dawned on me. My last egg was gone. The cupboard was bare. Etc etc. I would never ever have children. And that, we are told, from the moment we can absorb informa-tion, is the point of us, isn't it? Girls are there to make babies and, as women, to bear the load of caring for them.

I don't come from a long line of earth mothers. My mum has often been heard to joke that she doesn't like children except her own. (My brother and I have a standing gag that she doesn't like her own all of the time, either. That's not mean, that's just human. Nobody's likeable all of the time. Certainly not us.) My mum's mum – my nan – was a whole other kettle of fish. Let's just say she found life pretty unsatisfactory. To be fair, it probably was, as it was for most women of her age and class. Born into a large Catholic family in the 1920s to a black sheep mother, with a matriarch who majored on guilt, blame and shame and lavished it on my nan; married during the Second World War, worked in munitions. Her options were limited: leave school, get married, have kids, freeze vegetables (don't forget to blanch them), do the crossword, and think yourself lucky. Consequently, it's not unfair to say she didn't like anyone very much most of the time. Children, grandchildren, husband. She wasn't exactly a good advert for the heteronormative nuclear option.

Then there was my education. Or lack of it. The sole biology lesson I had at my huge small-town comprehensive in the late seventies was focused around reproduction. Sex was for making babies, wombs were for carrying them and periods were for flushing out those unused eggs and womb linings. Sperm swam and fought and battled like the macho little stormtroopers they were and any representation of intercourse we saw involved frogs. Contraception wasn't mentioned – apart from a memorable moment when our science teacher, Mrs Anthony-Roberts, showed us a five-minute film supposedly about sex and then, deeming it woefully uninformative, reduced the class to embarrassed titters by asking, 'Is it easier to put a condom on a cucumber or a sausage?' But the upshot was: sex is for procreation; otherwise, nice girls don't. (Boys, I guess, did what they always did: whatever they could get away with.) Menopause? Don't make me laugh.

Our paths were mapped out. Our families were mostly nuclear, our mums mostly didn't work until the youngest went to school (and then it was in part-time jobs that knocked off at three so they could get home before we did until we were old enough to legitimately be given our own key) and our dads mostly didn't know how to operate the cooker or the washing machine but were a whizz with the lawnmower and always took the bins out. I'm pretty sure not all the mums (or dads for that matter) liked it, but that was how it was, and as far as they were concerned it was how things were meant to be.

Back then, in my 13-year-old mind was a niggling thought that maybe it didn't have to be. That somewhere along the line, those roles could be overturned. And they can, to a lesser or greater extent. But you know what can't be overturned? Hormones.

'We may not define ourselves by our reproductive organs, whether we have children or not, but we are defined by them. Whatever your opinion about your role, your sex, your gender, your identity, your biology, your destiny, something is physically happening,' wrote Suzanne Moore in the *New Statesman* (her piece, 'There Won't Be Blood', is one of the best things I have ever read on the menopause and was a bit of a lifesaver when I was in the depths of despair – you should look it up[9]). That has never been clearer to me than when my hypothetical choice whether or not to have children was slowly but surely taken away. And I, a person who had studiously never defined myself by whether or not I had children – in fact I'd defined myself by almost anything but, which probably tells you all you need to know – was crying in the ladies because I could no longer have them.

I was picking away at this particular spot when I found a fascinating thread on American-Egyptian journalist and social commentator Mona Eltahawy's Twitter feed. The author of several books, including *The Seven Necessary Sins for Women and Girls*, Mona wrote that she was 52 and 'en route to menopause' and wanted to 'mark the change'. (Something so many women have said to me that I'm thinking menopause parties should be a thing.)

'I'm a child-free by choice cis woman,' she tweeted. 'I can imagine how much more difficult and challenging this change would be for a cis woman who had wanted children but could not for whatever reason, or non-binary and trans people going through it with such silence around it.'

The response was immediate. 'Mona, although I had no desire to have a child at 53 & was quite happy to finally be done with the menstrual cycle I found myself suddenly mourning it.' tweeted @violetflame16.

@kmcorby replied: 'I'm a little sad, too, at the loss of my fertility, even though I never had kids and never wanted them. Knowing you could bring forth life is still powerful.'

@violetflame16 agreed. 'Yes, it was the end of that powerful potential that I suddenly found myself slowly mourning. It took me by surprise – I had not expected that feeling at all. But it was the potential life-giving fertility that my body relinquished. I embrace the next phase wholeheartedly!

Further down the chain, I found this tweet from @schlatter_k. 'Turning 50 this year. Three years ago, my period got irregular for a few months and then – pouf – gone completely. As I never wanted children, my period was more of a nuisance than anything else. So I don't miss it one bit. On the contrary, it is extremely liberating.'

Of course, that's easy to say when your fertility, such as it was, has run its course in the prescribed fashion. But when you've experienced a premature or medical perimenopause (brought on by, for instance, hysterectomy or cancer treatment), it's a whole other matter.

Writer Allison Amend experienced early onset menopause at the age of 31. She wrote about it in a heart-rending article, 'Alone On A Path Shared By Many', in the *New York Times*. Like many women, she makes light of it, but it's no less traumatic for that. If you're feeling vulnerable about your own fertility, please take this as a Trigger Warning. 'When my cellphone rang ... I was already crying, driving to the airport to attend my aunt's funeral. My boyfriend had dumped me suddenly that morning via email ... When my doctor said, "I have bad news," I pulled over,' Allison wrote. '"You're in premature ovarian failure," she said. 'It's causing early onset menopause. I don't know how to tell you this: You won't be able to have children."'

Allison discovered she had previously undiagnosed Turner Syndrome (a chromosomal abnormality resulting from a prenatal mutation. Some of her cells were missing their second X chromosome). 'Once the tears stopped, I was filled with a deeper, duller sadness, like grief for a long-dead relative or childhood pet ... When I imagined my uterus and ovaries, I saw the citrus fruits they were inevitably compared to, but shrivelled and dry, wrinkled and useless. Who would want me now, a barren woman?'

If the language feels harsh, it is, intentionally so. It's, after all, the language society uses to describe the single, the child-free: spinster, barren, old maid. Yes, things have changed since Jane Austen's day, but the sentiment lingers. Add to that the language used to describe those on the other side of menopause – crone, hag, witch, old bag – and who wouldn't be depressed? It's bleak enough, without having to encounter it at 31.

'Still, I can't help but wonder about the lemonade that is supposed to result from these lemons,' Allison wrote later in her essay. 'The great man who comes to love me despite my failed ovaries and whose love I accept and return despite my feelings of inadequacy. I trust that some day it will no longer hurt to see pregnant friends and new babies, and that I won't feel like crying when people say, "You'll see, when you're pregnant". But for now, I miss the children I'll never give birth to as intensely as I miss the characters in a book after the last page is turned. I love them dearly, and yet they never existed.'

Lucy, 44, started her menopause early. She has one child and not having any more is one of the hardest things she's had to come to terms with. Or, perhaps, other people's expectations that she will have more ... 'I look younger than I am, and people are always asking me if I'm going to have a second one,' she says. 'It's not going to happen, but I find myself lying, saying I'd love to. I was 39 when I had my first child and I had such a traumatic birth. And yet it's all taboo ... I've just about gotten my head around talking about incontinence but this is just a whole new wave of shame.'

Writers Stella Duffy and Shelley Silas, who've been together for over twenty years, still had hoped to be parents after Stella was first diagnosed with breast cancer at 36. 'The day I was diagnosed with cancer was the day Shelley was going for our first insemination,' Stella recalls. 'So we put all that off for a bit. Shelley did get pregnant later that year but then miscarried and we never got pregnant again. I had five embryos made before chemo – this was 20 years ago and things have advanced, but back then chemo was 70 to 80 per cent likely to make you infertile – sadly they didn't survive.'

Stella is nothing if not glass half full. I hesitate to use the word 'inspiring', it's so exhausted, but in this case, given what she's been through it feels authentic. 'I'm genuinely glad to no longer have periods,' she insists. 'They were difficult and painful and uncomfortable and just all hard. And, once I found out I was unable to have kids, they were also really sad. And because we're gay there would be no happy accident. We had to choose to give up [on IVF] and that meant that was it, so it was really hard. Just sad. A reminder of the thing that wasn't happening.

'I remember people saying to me [when I started chemo], how are you going to cope with losing your hair? And I was like, "Oh my God, I'm losing my fertility, I don't give a fuck about my hair!"'

Shelley didn't go into menopause until far more recently. 'While I still had a uterus I kidded myself that the possibility of getting pregnant was very much alive,' she says, gently mocking herself in a way that becomes familiar if you spend enough time talking to women about their experience of the menopause. 'Even now, I have to remind myself that I no longer have one.

'I think it's really different for those of us who've tried and haven't had kids,' she continues. 'Once you're menopausal, it's like that's it, your chance has gone. It's the grief I didn't expect, and we're not given any help with that. I don't think anything can prepare you for it. It's such a physical thing. Menopause is not like just one day you stop having periods and that's that. It's so much more than that. It goes on and on and on.'

The day we speak, Tommy's National Centre for Miscarriage Research and Imperial College London publish research that found miscarriage may trigger PTSD. A third of women who miscarry subsequently suffer, it found, with some 25 per cent still suffering nine months later. Given that there are about 250,000 miscarriages in the UK each year – and a further 11,000 ectopic pregnancies – that's over 75,000, not exactly a small number of women. 'I think miscarriage and menopause are united,' says Shelley. 'They happen at different times of your life – but there's a massive expectation on us to just get over it because that's "what your body does".'

I'd expected that sense of loss and grief to be worse for those women who had always wanted children but been unable to have them. But Katy, 52, surprised me. 'I spent so much time grieving in my early forties after seven rounds of failed IVF,' she told me, 'that when menopause finally came, it wasn't a factor for me. Insomnia, weight gain, rage, anxiety, a sense of worthlessness, all those things, yes. But I had long since come to terms with the fact I would never be a biological mother. I'd made my peace with it.'

Motherhood is so loaded, so valued in our society – and yet not when it comes to attributing economic value to the emotional and human labour of caring. It's not surprising its curtailment is problematic. That said, the mothers I spoke to were as ambivalent about perimenopause as the non-mothers. One, a mum of four who confessed she gets broody every time she watches an episode of *One Born Every Minute*, said she couldn't quite believe there'd 'never be another baby through the door' and admitted she was still in denial about it, while another said two kids was more than enough and she couldn't wait to dispense with contraception. (The question as to why her partner hadn't shared that particular load didn't arise, as it didn't for many of the women I spoke to, but that's another book.) For several women, the end of fertility simply wasn't a big deal. They had other things to think about. Their lives had moved on. And then there were those who didn't want any more children, but still felt it keenly; it was the end of an era. An era that said something about them, regardless.

'There's a grief, isn't there?' actress Gillian Anderson, mother of three, and also a stepmother, said in an interview with *The Sunday Times Style*. 'I haven't quite got to the place where I don't have my eggs, but your body is going to mourn that, isn't it? I remember the very last time I breastfed and it was heartbreaking. I wept and wept through it.'

Marian Keyes recognised that sense of sorrow when I spoke to her for *The Shift* podcast. 'I had gone through the grief [of infertility] earlier, around the age of 40,' she told me, 'but I'd had three or four years to get used to it and as I got older I obviously knew it was less and less likely to happen, but the door was always open. There was always a chance. Then, around 48 I realised, "That's it. That really is it." It hit me anew.'

That struck a chord with me. I had just been reading author Iris Murdoch's famous description of menopause as the 'death of the womb' (melodramatic but also, you know, FACT) and an 'august and terrible pain', and it is. It's a kind of grief, a definite mournful regret, at least initially, but then, as that subsides, it's a sort of awakening. It made me wonder what, exactly, it is we are really mourning. Fertility? The children we never had? Or lost? Our youth? Certainly that's no small thing in a society as youth-focused as ours. Beauty? (Well, yes, assuming we had it in the first place. Ditto our elastic skin and firmer, more flexible body.) French model and music producer Caroline de Maigret, 44, author of *Older But Better, But Older*, told me that the French equivalent of the derogatory English 'old bag' is 'old skin'. More literally factual, and yet so brutal. And, yes, despite the fact that French men do age and presumably have similarly aged skin, it is only applied to women ... Plus ça change.) It's all of those things and, yet, none of them. What I think we're mourning, what we think is dying as our last egg departs, is hope; it's potential. And you know what, we're wrong. We might not have any eggs left but our potential is greater than ever.

It all goes back to Dr Jane Dickson's woman as 'pregnancy machine'. And we are – like it or not, consciously or not – 'a slave, with parts' until menopause comes and dismantles it all. Everything changes. Every single thing. And then, instead of being a person who can have babies (theoretically, if we're lucky, if we want them), we become a person who can't. A person in our own right. That's what I'm aiming for.

'If tomorrow women woke up and decided they really liked their bodies, just think how many industries would go out of business.'

Dr Gail Dines

4

GOOD MORNING, FLESH DUVET

Body image, body positivity and how to cope when the body formerly known as yours is replaced by one without a waist

One day, four, maybe five, years ago I woke up with a flesh duvet where my skin used to be. If you're pre-menopausal, you probably think I'm exaggerating, hamming it up for dramatic purpose, but I'm not. It literally happened that quickly. I went to bed averagely discontented with my body, as I did most nights, read too late, worried between the hours of 2 and 4am, and woke up at half past six ... middle-aged. As if, my brain having refused to accept that life might be moving on a little, my body had taken it into its own hands to help the process along. My skin had become squidgy, padded almost, with what felt like an inch of flesh beneath that definitely wasn't there before. You know when you poke your finger into a lump of dough and it gives, but doesn't automatically spring back up? That.

I admit, where my body is concerned, I have always had a few incy-wincy issues. Fewer now than ever. But still, if you're looking for someone well-balanced with a Positive Mental Attitude to write about how to get a grip on your body image post 50, I'm probably not your woman. I've been able to count calories since I was about seven (it was the seventies, every mum I knew spent the entire decade on a diet. Mind you, the same can be said for the eighties. And the nineties gave us heroin chic, so ...). But I'm getting ahead of myself.

This morning, the flesh duvet one, was the same as any other. The alarm went off. I ignored it. The cat-alarm went off, sat on my chest, bounced a bit (one of his back paws right on my nipple, the nubbly, painful bit. You know. How do they always manage to do that?), batted my nose with loosely flexed claws, put his face as close as he possibly could to mine and miaowed. Loudly. Repeatedly. Mouse breath.

In the face of cattrition I got up, grabbed my dressing gown from the floor so I didn't have to contend with my own nakedness this early in the morning and grumbled into the bathroom while the cat tried to herd me towards the stairs. In the bathroom I put on the really mean overhead lights, the ones designed to wake you the fuck up at 6am, turned the radio on and started going through my Monday-to-Friday cleanse, wash-off, moisturise, teeth-clean routine as I braced myself for the daily 'what shall I wear?' angst. Or, more truthfully, I weighed up what to wear from the four or five combos I alternate daily, despite having a wardrobe full of clothes. Then I pulled on some knickers, picked my bra up off the floor and it was as I reached round to do up the clasp that I noticed it.

Back fat.

I checked the bra strap wasn't all rucked up, spun the clasp round to the front and tried again. It did up, but even on the furthest set of hooks, the strap sank into my back, forcing little shelves of flesh over and under. Not that big of a deal in the scheme of things, except that it hadn't done that yesterday. The bra was the same, it hadn't shrunk overnight. It could only be the body that had changed. I squinted in the mirror. Something didn't look right. My knickers were tighter too. There was definite podge. And was my stomach – never exactly flat or firm, just sort of stomachy – a bit wobblier? I poked it. It did that dough thing. So I poked the back of my upper arm, my thigh in several places, and my back, right where my bra had displaced some of it. Then I had a go at the flesh under my chin. Let's call a spade a spade: my double chin.

WTAF? I went back into the bedroom. Trailed by a livid cat.

No, no, no, don't do it. DO NOT DO IT.

'Have I put on weight?'

Too late. Groggily, Jon rolled over and pushed himself up on his elbows. 'I can't see from here.'

Uh-oh. Quit while you're still just about ahead. I didn't. I stepped nearer.

'Maybe. A bit.' He shrugged, and crashed back down on to the mattress. (Never marry an honest man, that's my advice. And novelists are worse. Clinically objective.)

I stormed back into the bathroom, grabbed yesterday's jeans and thrust my legs into them. Of *course* I hadn't put on weight overnight. Don't be ridiculous. Pulled them up. Oh. Turns out they agreed with him.

Honest to God it was as if the fat fairies had come during the night and coated me with an extra layer of insulation. Head to toe. Although, maybe not toes. Or fingers. But the rest. It wasn't huge, but it was definitely noticeable. Like a sudden full-body premenstrual bloat. And like premenstrual bloat, I told myself, it would be gone tomorrow. Or if not tomorrow, then the next day or the next. But then premenstrual bloat is just that. Premenstrual. It goes when the period comes. But this time there was no period. Instead, as the days passed, the flesh duvet seemed to be bedding in; like relatives at Christmas who outstay their welcome, it made itself at home and started slowly but surely to become a permanent annoyance.

Clothes that fitted perfectly well yesterday no longer did up quite so smoothly today. Clothes I had worn day in, day out for weeks on end no longer suited me. If not overnight then certainly over the course of just a few weeks, my trusty uniform abandoned me. I looked in the mirror and no longer looked quite like me any more.

It wasn't about the weight so much as the way my clothes fit. I don't know how much I weigh – although I can hazard a guess – but the scales and I parted ways in my early twenties when, after a decade of what we now call severely disordered eating, I realised that they had a disproportionate influence on my mood. If I was ever going to get even the slightest grip on my body image, the scales had to go in the bin. They've been there ever since. But freeing myself from the tyranny of the scales has not released my self-esteem from being hinged to my size. I mean, who really needs scales when you're so attuned to the fit of your clothes? True, they can't swing by four pounds overnight like scales can as a result of water retention, or particularly heavy knickers. Or I thought they couldn't, but it turns out menopause had news for me.

Given my erratic history, I should have paid more attention to the changes that might be wrought on my body by the end of oestrogen. But I didn't. I noticed when other women's bodies changed – because that's what we do, isn't it? Look at each other's bodies and judge ourselves in comparison; and one of us is inevitably found wanting. That's what being a woman is, being found wanting. But I didn't think that would happen to me. Oh, bless my naivety. Because that's what it was: the end of oestrogen. With hindsight, it's another thing that should have been blindingly obvious but wasn't. Puberty is accompanied by an oestrogen surge that brings, to a varying degree, breasts, waist, hips and periods, not necessarily in that order. For me, breasts not so much, but the hips were plentiful and so I also had a waist. Menopause is the anti-puberty if you like: away goes the oestrogen, away goes the blood and with it away goes the waist (and the skin elasticity). I had longed to see the back of that waist (and the childbearing hips that went with it), but I'd anticipated the hips shrinking, not the waist expanding.

Of all the women I spoke to, just one said she was happy with her body. Out of more than 50. Regardless of age, race, class, weight, geography or sexuality. Almost every single one thought she could stand to lose half a stone. Or a stone. Or a dress size. (Karen, 50, sometimes a 12, sometimes a 14, wisely described dress size as a 'slippery slope'. I think the ever-shifting size 12 (or whatever) is practically gaslighting.) Those who said they were 'accepting' of their bodies also described an immense amount of work to get there and stay there. Society has conditioned us to know what we *should* look like and we look in the mirror and invariably find ourselves wanting. My own obsessions have roved around my body as I've aged, starting with bum and thighs as a young teenager, taking in boobs (too small), stomach (too big), chin (too many) and now stomach again, with arms a close second. And now, in the gym this morning, doing stomach curls with added weights (ouch), I noticed it in the mirror. There was no getting away from it. My neck. I clocked it, I looked again, I WTFed it. And then I thought, you know what, I already feel bad about my stomach and my thighs. I refuse to feel bad about my neck. ('I will not let society bully me into having an issue with my arms!' raged Helen, 45. We were talking about sleeves ...)

'Susie Orbach's *Fat is a Feminist Issue* was seminal for me, so was Naomi Wolf's *The Beauty Myth*,' says Kate Spicer. They were for me, too. Though I would also throw in the lesser-known *The Hungry Self* by Kim Chernin. All three books have been on my shelves since the late eighties/early nineties; revisited so many times they're dog-eared, their spines cracked and pages loose from repeated reading. In my early twenties I inhaled their teachings. I felt the innate rightness of what they had to say about the impact of misogyny on the way I felt about my body, how I had internalised a male gaze that was all about tits and arse, and a fashion industry that dictated that a woman's body should not be so present as to get in the way of the clothes. And yet, knowing all that, I've still spent most of my life counting calories. And working in magazines that covered fashion. And being slightly obsessed with clothes.

Kate's the same, although she probably resorted to a more colourful array of methods than binge-starve-vomit to stop the weight going on. 'I think our generation – Gen X, the one that's shifting now – was brought up with a fairly narrow idea of what we should look like,' she says. 'I *know* that. But, still, I never want to be over ten stone. Up to about ten stone I can carry it. Nine stone I feel comfortable in a bikini, ten stone I feel comfortable in clothes. Over that it starts making me feel a bit uncomfortable.'

She looks me in the eye. 'For you and me, it was a constant internal battle.' I feel seen. We have never discussed our respective eating problems in any kind of detail, but I guess it takes one to know one. We worked together briefly in the nineties on a now long-defunct magazine called *Minx*, when we were both around 30, and you don't have to share a desk for too long to get a sense of your desk mate's hang-ups. The job was a thankless one. I only just survived my stint as editor by swimming at the pool across the road from the office at 7.30 every morning. Like most of my life, I thought I wasn't good enough, which manifested as thinking I was overweight. I wasn't. How I felt had nothing to do with my weight. I know that now, but I still don't always pay attention to it. It makes me sad, the time I spent worrying about my body and how it didn't look the way I thought it should. The days, weeks, months, even years, trying to force myself to fit some imaginary ideal when, to paraphrase Nora Ephron, I wish I'd spent most of my twenties in a bikini.

For a while, menopause brought all those feelings flooding back. The sense of inadequacy that found an outlet in my relationship with my body. It was exactly like being 13, 14, 15 again. The internal rage at life's injustices, the explosions of temper, the sense of impotence, that nothing was within your own control. 'Living with you the last couple of years has been like living in the eye of a storm,' Jon said. More likely, I think now, it was like living with a teenage girl in the midst of puberty. All unfocused rage and self-loathing bubbling over at inopportune moments.

My problems with food peaked, the first time, at 15. The oestrogen had kicked in, everything was out of control, subconsciously self-starvation was the only way to regain it. Yes, the dumpy ginger freckly kid I'd always been became a thin girl with a much vaunted inner thigh gap, while the scales hovered around seven stone. And yes, I still thought I was fat. But that wasn't what it was about. It never is. It was about owning something, taking charge. It was about me.

Is it any wonder that, as my body spiralled back out of control in my late forties, I started, briefly, seeking new ways to control it? It's increasingly common for perimenopausal women to experience a resurgence of past eating disorders. In the US, 13 per cent of women over 50 are believed to engage in disordered eating[10] whereas 3.5 per cent of 'mid-life women' (i.e. women over 40) in the UK are believed to have a full-blown eating disorder, over half of whom are first-timers.[11] The number of women seeking help for disordered eating in their late forties and beyond has risen by a startling 42 per cent in the last decade.[12]

I'm aware as I type this how much I and many women, and not just of my generation, have internalised the model of female attractiveness first peddled by the society I grew up in – a seventies world of heatwave summers, the F-Plan, the South Beach Diet and Jane Fonda workouts; a world where it wasn't frowned on to have a well-worn calorie guide in the kitchen junk drawer and eat bare Ryvita for lunch five days a week. (Now, of course, we eat rice cakes and avocado and drink bulletproof coffee and do the 16:8 daily fast ... but we're not dieting, we're clean eating our way to wellness, so that's OK.)

No matter how evolved I tell myself I am, more than 30 years on I still think I can stand to lose seven pounds. (Actually, postmenopause it's more like a stone.) But emotionally, I have moved on. When the oestrogen went and the pounds went on, it ultimately wasn't the weight I was most worried about, it was my identity. Yes, there was the whole waist thing, the loss of flexibility, the waning strength and the back ache, the occasional stoop and the involuntary groaning when I got out of bed. But more than that, it was the state of the inside of my head. And while we all know exercise can make us stronger, fitter and all that, it's our mental health that needs it most.

When times have been really tough, I have always instinctively fallen back on exercise. It's like my body knows what to do even when my head doesn't. I'm not sporty, I'm hopeless at team sports, I was always picked last for games. I couldn't climb, or back flip or vault or cartwheel. I run at the pace of a snail. The only thing I was ever any good at was swimming. And I didn't even take my feet off the bottom till I was ten. By the time I was 13, I was swimming, ferociously, obsessively, competitively. I wasn't the best in the team by far, but it gave me focus. I was good at something other than English homework and I got up most mornings at 6.30am to train with the local club (my poor parents). It didn't last long, I ditched it when I was 15 and started to care more about my hair frizzing and getting a boyfriend than being the fastest swimmer in town and winning a medal. In other words, right around the time oestrogen kicked in. Can't help feeling there's a connection there.

It happened again when I edited *Minx*. I swam my way to sanity. This time, in the midst of perimenopause, telling myself I was too busy to take time out for me, I tried to walk my way to sanity instead. I walked everywhere. And as I walked, head down, earphones in, ploughing through audiobook after audiobook, I embarked on a battle with myself to become a person who didn't care. A person who had no fucks left to give for waists and hips and dress sizes. 'Who cares whether you've got a waist?' I told myself. 'This is me, take it or leave it.' For a while, I was almost convinced.

I got a Fitbit and within weeks exercise only counted if the Fitbit registered it. I went from 10,000 steps a day to 12,000 to 15,000. I started walking up and down stairs repeatedly before I went to bed, to get my steps up. But it wasn't the answer. Walking is medicine in its own right. It gets you out of the house, it clears your head, it saves you bus fares, but walking alone doesn't make you stronger or more flexible. I still creaked when I got up and sometimes when I sat down. My knees were rickety. My back still ached. Far from being able to touch my toes, I could barely reach my knees. And it certainly didn't reach my middle. My face didn't look 50, I was sure of it, but my body certainly felt it.

At the same time I, subconsciously or otherwise, stopped wearing jeans and spent an entire summer shrouded in a blue smock dress from Other Stories and my faithful Converse. Walking clothes, I told myself. Hiding clothes would have been more truthful. The bigger I felt, the smaller I tried to be. My self-esteem, always precarious, went through the floor. My therapist Tessa, who at that point I'd been seeing nearly 18 months, noticed. 'You don't have to just put up with it, you know,' she said. I glared at her balefully. Realising as I did so that here was a woman somewhere in her fifties who looked her age, but also looked great on it. Tall, strong, slim. 'Weights,' she said. 'You want to be strong and fit, to have a body to live the rest of your life in, you want weights.'

I logged it, but dismissively, and we went our separate ways for summer break; she to wherever therapists go in August, me to a Greek island where I bikini-dodged for 14 days. Recently I found some pictures from that holiday; I'm wearing a black one-piece and a big sunhat, spine curved, shoulders hunched protectively around my body at the edge of a clear blue pool, my posture ageing me more than my body ever could.

'Weights,' said an article a few weeks later in *The Times* by health and beauty journalist Alice Hart-Davis. It was about a gym in London called The Clock. Founded by Zana Morris, it boasted a 15-minute daily programme that guaranteed results in 12 days. It wasn't cheap. And only promised results if you followed its high-fat diet simultaneously. Plus it was expensive. Too expensive to justify. I filed it away.

'Weights,' said my friend Anna who had done the programme at that same gym. 'You'll never look back.'

I cracked. My therapy had just finished and I convinced myself that I could justify spending what would have been the cost of four weeks' therapy on the 12-session programme. The first time I set foot in that gym I was terrified. I had learnt the hard way to fear sporty people at school and the idea of voluntarily submitting to their pincers and their scales and their weight programmes terrified me. I made them cover the screen of the scales before I stood on them. To this day I don't know what I weighed, but after various calculations and some uncomfortable manoeuvres with a set of calipers, it transpired my BMI was over 30. In short, I was technically obese; fat on the inside. I'm a lapsed vegetarian, so the high-fat diet wasn't easy. For the 3 weeks it took to complete 12 sessions, I subsisted mainly on tuna and Greek yoghurt. Oh, and no booze. Let's face it, on that diet who wouldn't lose weight? But already I was more interested in the growth of my muscles and how my body felt than the weight loss, which I was told would have been seven pounds if you took off the muscle I'd gained. I was hooked. I felt great, and for the next year I devoted three lunchtimes a week (I even made sure I took lunch hours – what a revelation that was) and ate a helluva lot of protein. Over that time, my BMI dropped to 23 and I lost another seven pounds. I still don't know where that means I ended up on the scales. But more importantly, for the first time in my 50-odd years I understood that exercise had as much to do with my mind as my body, and 35 years after Maths GCSE I worked out the input versus output equation where calories are concerned. I understood them, at last, as a unit of energy. I know. It was a revelation! Muscles began to form where previously there hadn't been any, the low-level back ache I'd lived with for more than 20 years abated, my posture improved and my lung capacity began to deepen. Slowly, my waist returned(ish). If anything, my body image is better than it's ever been. And yet my body definitely isn't. Weight training transformed my attitude to my body. It flicked a switch in my head that taught me to be grateful for what it could do for me, rather than how it looked. (Although I'm still not free of that and probably never will be.) And crucially, for the first time since perimenopause kicked in, and probably far longer, I felt strong.

'My body is what makes me realise I'm old,' says Juliet, 50. 'It breaks more than it used to. It takes longer to fix than it used to. I can't just bash it around and know that it will recover. I've also had this massive revelation that food is not about calories, it's about feeding your body. So now I think about food as something that makes me strong, rather than something that makes me fat or thin. I just want to feel well and it wasn't until I was 48 or 49 that I properly got that lightbulb moment.'

Juliet isn't the only one who felt her body was ageing her. 'What really hit me when I became menopausal was this rapid weight gain and the loss of a waist, which I'd always had,' says Genevieve, 57. 'I've always looked young in the face but my body was trying to turn me into an old woman.'

Bestselling novelist and screenwriter Jojo Moyes became an exercise devotee in her late forties. It started with boxing and she now runs several times a week and has a personal trainer. At 50, her body – and her attitude to it – has changed beyond all recognition. 'I had a frozen shoulder for 18 months, which is a classic thing for women of a certain age (if you believe in Chinese medicine it's also to do with carrying the burden of life). I remember my best friend saying to me "you are literally hunched like an old woman, you need to straighten up". I started boxing because I wanted to improve my shoulder strength and core strength. I was a very weedy kid, I was never athletic, hopeless at ball sports. But

75

it turns out, to my great joy, that hitting is the thing I'm really good at!

'I like feeling fit. I'm really enjoying having muscles that I didn't have and feeling like my back doesn't hurt all the time. What's really clear to me is that if I keep doing all the exercise and I keep running, then stuff doesn't hurt. It's as simple as that. I can eat all the chocolate I like and I can have the curry on a Friday night, but if I stop for a few weeks it all turns to Jabba the Hut. Strength is absolutely key. I don't care what size my jeans are but I don't want to have problems with my knees and my hips. Like it or not, this is the downside of being this age, you have to use it or lose it. I look better and I'm fitter now than I was at 40. That's quite a nice thing, if I'm honest.'

Like Jojo, Karen, also 50, feels better about her body now than she has since her twenties. 'I started exercising regularly six years ago, when my dad was diagnosed with cancer and I needed to ensure I was healthy enough to take him to chemo and dialysis 90 minutes away 3 times a week. It ended up being something that contributed as much to my mental health as physical. Since I've become more curious about what my body can do strength and fitness wise, I've gone from 34 per cent to 20 per cent body fat and now I focus on strength and challenging myself without comparing myself to others. No amount of effort has changed the lack of tone around my stomach and I'm at peace with it. Something I wasn't when I was younger.'

However your body image stacks up, the mind–body equation is key. Kate, also 50 (I'm spotting a theme ...): 'I've started open water swimming in the summer and in the winter I go to the Serpentine, swim 15 metres and then get out! It's amazing. When you get in cold water, all the blood rushes to your organs to protect them because it thinks you're going to freeze to death and when you get out it rushes to your skin. But when it goes to your organs it picks up loads of goodness and extra juicy bits and then it flushes your body with all this good shit so it's fucking healthy for you. It's good for your mood and it doesn't cost any money. I go in feeling one way and ten seconds later I come out feeling totally different.'

'I have always understood the importance of movement to balance my emotional state,' says Nahid de Belgeonne, 52, founder of The Human Method (a form of yoga designed to help those fatigued from our always-on culture). 'I started running when I wanted to leave home. I started kickboxing when I wanted to leave my first husband. I started to practise yoga when I left a stressful job and big income with no plans ... movement really is medicine to me.'

One thing that really struck me when I was researching this book was how rarely the weight gain and changing body shape that menopause brings was confronted head-on. Yes, it came up obliquely in the context, say, of the erosion of femininity some women experience (I definitely feel less 'womanly' but then I was never a girly girl to start with). But the books I read hardly mentioned it. That was in stark contrast to the women I spoke to. For them, a change in weight and body shape was part and parcel of their loss of confidence and self-esteem, often going hand in hand with confusion, anxiety and plummeting self-confidence. Time and again they told me their body image was at an all-time low, whether they had spent their lives on a diet, or hadn't given their weight a second thought until they hit their forties, and then boom. For many it was worse even than when they were a teenager. Combined with their fears that they were about to be consigned to the dustbin of life, it was just one more thing that confirmed their growing sense that they were either no longer worthy of taking up space or vain and shallow for caring; either way it made them feel somehow less. Instead of judging women for feeling bad about their bodies, shouldn't we be addressing the core problem: the society that makes us feel we are only as good as we look in the first place?

'I've kept a rein on my dress size throughout my life out of pure vanity,' says Paula, 49. 'I won't accept that being menopausal is going to make me bigger, I'm going to fight that bastard. I'm more healthy now than in my twenties. I consider what I eat.'

Jenny, 48, was, in her own words, 'a complete rake in my teens and twenties ... My body shape never concerned me because I was society's desired shape.' Now, two stone heavier, but still a slim size 14, she's on a diet, hoping to lose a stone. 'I haven't told a soul because I feel judged, scorned,' she admits, 'I just want to scream. If I'm in charge of my body and I'm doing this for me, what's the damn problem?'

There's an uncomfortable dichotomy at work here: on the one hand, women are branching out, pushing boundaries, forcing conversations in all kinds of areas – body positivity, gender neutrality, mental health awareness, sexual harassment, pay parity – and ending relationships that no longer work for us, leaving jobs that are making us ill. We are taking less shit and being more overtly ourselves, whatever shape that may take, than ever before. On the other hand, here we are, just as likely to be judged on our dress size as we ever were. Perhaps more importantly, just as likely to judge ourselves on it.

Spend five minutes on Instagram and tell me you don't come away confused. Should you be taking semi-naked selfies and loving your cellulite, as the body positivity movement tells us, or should you be juice-fasting your way to a 'bikini' body? The one thing that is consistent on both sides of the perfection divide is the judgement. The pressure to do it right, look right, *be* right. Who the fuck knows what constitutes right? Not me. But, as ever, where women's bodies are concerned, there's an awful lot of *should* going on. And somewhere in the middle are hundreds of thousands, make that millions, of women who don't love themselves, much as they wish they could, who don't have the confidence to stick two fingers up to society, and yet for whom the pressure to do just that is as overpowering as the pressure to lose that stone. It becomes yet another thing we're doing wrong. The upshot? Loving ourselves becomes just another thing on the to-do list. Don't know about you, but I'm exhausted by it.

'I find body positivity overwhelming,' says Clare, 48. 'Another thing that as a woman I'm supposed to embrace and support. I would just settle for feeling confident in how I look and dress.'

Jenny is by her own admission 'ambivalent'. 'I think it's fantastic that women of all shapes and sizes have got more confidence to wear what they want, if they want and when they want,' she says. 'That makes me want to punch the air. However, I personally do want to lose some weight. I'm conscious that if I don't, in another decade I could be another stone heavier and I don't want that. I can tell physically that I don't feel as great as I have, so this extra weight on me is obviously taking a bit of a toll physically as well as psychologically. But I don't feel I can admit that.'

Helen, 45, feels at a place of acceptance with her own body, which 'feels more achievable'. 'I don't think body positivity or body acceptance is mainstream, though,' she adds. 'I think most women feel like they need to be thinner. It's so ingrained.'

'While the body positivity movement celebrates all bodies that spill over the waistband of what is currently acceptable, it fails to illuminate the reasons why so many people have such bitter and violent relationships with their bodies to begin with,' wrote Eva Wiseman in a column advocating body neutrality in the *Observer*. 'The reasons so many people hate their bodies go deeper than a Dove ad can explain, and they are good reasons – they may not be correct, they may be horrific and mean and based in decades of well-funded sexism, but they are logical, and they were taught to us young. So the impact of enforcing body positivity on people who, under their skin, know there are rational reasons they have sex with the lights off, or fear exercising in public, or click on Instagram links to cosmetic surgeons in Turkey, or have been on diets since they were 12, can feel like two trucks crashing in their throat ... The effect, then, was a feeling of isolation, and a doubling of guilt. Guilt both for living in a body that doesn't fit and for wanting to change it.'

The endless pressure to be something you're not makes Marian Keyes 'feckin' livid'. 'The weight gain of menopause!' she exclaims. 'I wish someone would say, give it up, let it go, this is your size now. This is what it SHOULD be.'

It feels like for many women, permission to give yourself a break is key; to reach a place of 'proud ambivalence', as Wiseman puts it. To stop wasting our energy worrying whether we're wearing the wrong thing, looking the wrong way and doing the wrong thing, and start recognising who we are and what we – and so many other women, be they on the beach, in the supermarket queue, in the coffee shop – have achieved. OK, so we shouldn't need to look outside ourselves for acceptance, we all know that. But if, in this moment of intense disruption and dislocation, we don't feel able to find it within – and perhaps never have – and there's not a chance in hell of society giving it to us, maybe we need to look to the people/women we surround ourselves with, in life and online; the markers and language we use around this stage of our life and what lies beyond. We are here, we are healthy, we have bodies that have done amazing things. OK, so they might not be perfect by society's standards, but they are ours, so let's help each other celebrate them.

'There's a reason why 40, 50 and 60 don't look the way they used to and it's not because of feminism or better living through exercise, it's because of hair dye.'

Nora Ephron

5

HAIR IS EVERYTHING

The politics of going grey. Or not going grey

I'm not sure how old I was when I started going grey, but I know how old I was when people started pointing it out: 47. (I say people, but really I mean one people. One was plenty.) There I was, happily bobbing along, still thinking of myself as The Girl With The Big Red Hair™, a role I'd happily fulfilled since my late teens, and it turned out it was no longer true. Well, the big hair bit was, but the 'red' and the 'girl' not so much. (Not that I wasn't already fully aware that 'girl' was chancing it.) I was recruiting for the first few jobs for what was to become The Pool, and had arranged to meet a Cool Young Woman in a coffee shop near what laughingly passed for our office. After having to front out all the tech geeks and the money men who couldn't quite work out what the point of me was, I was finding all the Cool Young Women I was meeting a bit terrifying but also blissfully refreshing in their confidence and, yes, entitlement. (Why shouldn't they be entitled? All the tech and finance bros were.)

I knew little about this particular CYW other than that I had enjoyed some pieces she'd written and 'people' raved about her. She was fast, she was funny, she was adaptable, she had written – I was reliably informed – for 'everyone' (some of them all in one day, so the internet goes ...). And, best of all, we might even be able to afford her. The CYW rushed in a few minutes late, Lycra-clad, bike helmet flying, and I bought her a coffee. As I bum-shuffled back on to the high bench clearly not designed for people who are 5 foot 4, she looked at me and beamed. 'I love your hair,' she gushed. 'You're so brave going grey.'

Oh.

'Th-thanks,' I managed to mumble. And then my mind went blank. It wasn't that I minded her saying it, she meant it as a compliment. I'm sure she did. I was 'brave', after all. And that's a good thing, isn't it? (Hang on, it's *hair*. There's nothing brave about it.) It was that I truly hadn't realised I was going grey until that moment.

It was a long 45 minutes. Mainly because, vain creature that I am, I couldn't get the comment out of my head. I'm going grey. I'm SO going grey that complete strangers comment on it. IN JOB INTERVIEWS.

Back in the office, I peered at my roots in the loo. She was right. I was going grey. And when I examined it further, it was worse at the front, and it wasn't just my roots. When I lifted my hair on the right-hand side, it turned out I had a large grey patch – heavy at the roots, but reaching all the way to the ends – on exactly the spot where I'd hit my head in that car crash at university. (I didn't know, at the time, that this was a thing. Apparently it is.)

It was like someone had told me I was no longer Sam. My very Sam-ness had been taken away. Removed. Leached out. I'm a bit embarrassed by the way I (over)reacted. It's just hair FFS. And my hair was no different to the way it was the day before. The only difference was that CYW had woken me up to the fact that what I'd blithely been thinking of as slightly faded ginger was actually grey. It wasn't her fault. (But, really, in a JOB INTERVIEW?!)

It took me a long time to embrace my hair. At school I was freckly and swotty, with huge wavy ginger hair, in a school of

1,500 kids where you could count the gingers on one hand. No insult passed without reference to it. I'm only grateful I'd left school by the time the word minger was invented. I looked like nothing so much as Barb from *Stranger Things*, minus the glasses. Things only began to change when, at 15, I started growing it. Apart from a brief diversion to black via student gothdom and an ill-advised break-up bob in my late teens, I've had big red hair ever since. Big red hair is a thing. When I was talking to writer Stella Duffy about her premature menopause brought on by cancer, she looked at me meaningfully when she talked about losing her hair as a result of chemo. 'You know, the whole long red hair thing ...' she said. And we both nodded, in silent communion. Gingers united. (Stella had it worse than me, she was called 'period head' at school.) It's the stick they beat you with at school – or one of them, and then you wrestle the stick away from them. You own the stick. You make it yours.

Anyway, I was so freaked out by the whole grey thing that the next time I saw my long-time hairdresser Adam Reed, I tentatively suggested it might be time to start dyeing. He was so shocked he actually dropped the bit of my hair he was holding and took a step back. 'Say that again.'

I said it again.

He laughed. 'You? *You* want to dye your hair?'

Yes, me.

To be fair, he had a point. I've knocked back all attempts to dye my hair as long as he's known me, and he started cutting my hair when I was editor of *Cosmopolitan*. And one of the many things I love about Adam is that he has never done that hairdresser thing of trying to make me cut it off/dye it/whatever. (Why do hairdressers do that? If I had a tenner for everyone who'd accosted me in the street offering to chop it off, I'd have a lot of tenners.)

'Why not?' I asked. 'The grey is really starting to show.'

84

He put on his best strict-dad face. 'Sam,' he said. 'Even if you needed it – which I don't think you do, but obviously it's up to you – there's no way you'll sit still long enough.' He proceeded to reel off all the processes that an initial dye on hair of my length (which is so long, I can hook it up under my arm and still have a couple of inches to spare) would need, and then moved on to the three–four weekly maintenance appointments required to keep the roots covered.

He had a point. I'm pretty low maintenance where grooming is concerned. Too busy, I tell myself. Too lazy, is probably nearer the truth. I'm also fair-skinned, so where for years I hated my non-existent eyebrows and eyelashes, now-menopausal-me loves them. I haven't grown a moustache, I don't have the random wiry hair problem (yet). I don't wax, I don't dye, I don't thread, I don't do anything much except cleanse and moisturise moisturise moisturise, and go to the hairdresser once every three (OK, six) months. So was I really going to spend whole days in foils and then go back every few weeks and spend another three hours getting my roots done? I don't spend that much time on maintenance in a whole year. And as for the cost ...

'Also,' Adam said, sitting on his spinny stool, dad-face to the max. '*Why?*'

Why? It was a question I should have asked myself before I bothered him with it. Why did I freak out when an innocent bystander commented on my nascent grey? Why was my immediate, unfettered reaction to dye it? And why, now, five years later, when my hair is a weird concoction of reds, blondes, beiges, browns and greys that are entirely – for better or worse – natural, am I seriously considering dyeing the whole lot silver?

Identity, that's why. The hair itself is just a side issue.

I'd been asking the wrong question all along. The question should have been: who am I, if I'm not The Girl With The Big

Red Hair? And why, after everything I've done, do I still feel, Samson-like, that it all rests in my hair? The truth is, my ginger has gone – or it's well on the way out – and I'm having to dig deep to discover who I am now it's not there.

When I was about 25, Jon and I went to Paris for the weekend. Sitting on the metro, on the way back from the flea market at Clignancourt, I noticed an old French woman staring at me across the carriage. As the train pulled into a station, she started taking tentative, evidently painful, steps towards me. Drawing level, she stopped so we were almost toe-to-toe. 'You have beautiful hair,' she said, putting out her hand to touch it. 'I used to have hair like this.' She was chic, petite, attractive, 80ish, maybe more. Her hair was a pretty grey, almost white, pulled tight to her head in a chignon. 'It's beautiful,' she said, almost mournfully. She looked back longingly as she stepped on to the platform. Then she was gone. Am I that woman now? Well, no. But I'm beginning to know how she felt.

My hair is – or was – slightly what I imagine having a baby bump is like. A touch magnet. So while it was invasive, it didn't faze me at all that a complete stranger stroked it on the Paris metro. Old ladies in particular often came up to me gazing longingly at my hair. It was once offered a part in an 'Italian film' when Jon and I were in the French House pub in Soho, as long as I accompanied the elderly 'director' to Venice immediately. (No, I didn't go. Can't help wondering, though ...) I was good for free Guinness all night in Camden on St Patrick's Day. I had that sort of hair. My hair was more popular than me.

I treated it abysmally. I rarely had it cut, I washed it every two weeks if it was lucky, I never blow-dried it and I certainly never brushed or combed it. I took it for granted. I was the classic bad boyfriend. And now it's gone. (Well, some of it has.) Neglected and taken for granted for decades, my huge wavy hair that grew like wildfire now tends towards rats' tails or frizz. It's prone to

split ends. My skin got moisturised religiously, twice daily, sometimes more. My hair ... not so much. Is it any wonder that like the
rest of me it's ageing?

'Hair is everything,' said Phoebe Waller-Bridge in the episode
of *Fleabag* where she berates the hairdresser who makes her
sister, played by Sian Clifford, look 'like a pencil'. 'We wish it
wasn't, so we could actually think about something else occasionally. But it is. It's the difference between a good day and a bad
day. We're meant to think that it's a symbol of power, that it's a
symbol of fertility. Some people are exploited for it and it pays
your fucking bills. Hair is everything.'

That scene broke the internet. And it broke the internet
because it's true. And you know which bit is particularly true
if you're going grey: 'It's a symbol of power, it's a symbol of
fertility.' Oh, hey, old grey wispy/wiry lady, do you want a
symbol of your infertility and powerlessness on your head?
Not so much, thanks. Because that's what it boils down to.
Not only do we carry our identity around on our heads, we
internalise all the things we think it says about us. Look me in
the eye and tell me you don't think of yourself as a blonde, or
a brunette or a redhead, or indeed grey and proud, or someone who changes their hair colour as often as their clothes,
and have never ever used hair colour or type or style as a
means by which to judge others. We use it to tell the world
what we want it to think about us – whether it's gamine,
cropped, shaved, natural afro, pre-Raphaelite, shampoo-ad
silky, peroxide blonde, pink, Louise Brooks bob, extensions,
wild, neat ... Whatever we do with it, it's our calling card. And
what the world tells us it thinks about grey hair (specifically
on women) is that – unless you're 25 and hashtag granny hair,
in which case, go you, style statement – it's not going to
bother thinking about us at all.

'For the same reasons that our hair seems to symbolise who
we are as individuals, it also symbolises where – or if – we fit

in society,' says Rose Weitz, author of *Rapunzel's Daughters: What Women's Hair Tells Us about Women's Lives*. 'Because hair is so invested with meaning, it becomes a marker of our very identities. We may be judged by our hair in school, by friends, in the workplace, and in romantic relationships. It's not surprising that some focus on their hair as a means of controlling their identity and maintaining or changing their place in the world.'

The upshot? 'Even if, in the abstract, we think we look all right with grey hair,' she says, 'we nonetheless feel we are losing our "real selves" if we no longer have our "real hair colour".'

In the same book, she quotes author John Molloy as saying that 'women with grey hair are considered over the hill and old by the majority of business people.' Admittedly that was in 1996 and things have, thankfully, moved on. A little. When I used to commute daily to London there was a woman I saw regularly who had the most spectacular thick silver bob. It was the only thing about her that stood out. Otherwise, she was just another woman somewhere in her early fifties, in a skirt suit and low heels, carrying too many bags. One evening, as we queued to get off the carriage, I complimented her on it. She laughed. 'Tell that to the men I work with.' She worked, she told me, for an American bank and spent most of her time in New York. 'They don't know what to do with me there,' she said. 'They call me "the grey lady". Grey is obviously their shorthand for old.'

I'd like to slightly amend that statement: grey is obviously their shorthand for old, *when appended to women*. (Men, as we all know, are not 'grey men' but 'silver foxes' ...) It's hardly surprising then that we're so conflicted about letting our grey go. Look at the UK parliament and tell me how many women you see with a head of grey hair. Off the top of my head, I can think of one, Theresa May ... (I'm saying nothing.) US Congress? Business is the same (with the honourable exception of the statement grey of the President of the European Central Bank, Christine Lagarde). Now do the same exercise for men. Excuse me if I don't wait while you do the calculations.

I truly couldn't care less what colour anyone's hair is, each to their own, do what feels right for you, but as with all things, it's not just a you issue. If only it was. It's a feminist issue. And I admit there's a little bit of that going on for me. Why should we have to put ourselves through all this aggro when, out there, men with grey hair, salt-and-pepper hair, and no hair at all are bigger, bolder, more prominent – more promoted – than ever before. How come, as Lena asked earlier, men are silver foxes, while women who go grey are just … old.

This was definitely a factor when, aged a not-remotely-old 42, fashion director Anna Murphy decided to ditch the hair dye and let her trademark curly dark brown fade to grey. 'I came to realise, for me hair was a feminist issue. I was getting annoyed about the whole fandango. Did I really have to pretend my hair was something other than what it was, to look my best, to feel attractive, when men didn't do the same?' she wrote in *The Times*.

If you want to make yourself nauseous with rage, google 'hair rules' or 'hair age' or, God forbid, 'grey hair' or 'hair over 40'. The outcome is pretty much the same. Assuming you've got other things to do than lose hours of your life that you'll never get back down a Google hole, here are just some of the things the internet/media/self-appointed experts are pretty adamant you should not do with your hair if you are over 40:

Don't keep it long. Especially not 'cat lady' long. (Oops)
Don't keep the same hairstyle you've always had.
Don't go too dark.
Don't keep it all one length.
Don't go shorter in the front than the back – eh?

Don't part it in the 'wrong' place.
Don't 'wear' your hair too big.
... Or too flat.

How's your stamina? In the market for a few more gems?

> If you were worrying that long hair makes women over 40 look like mutton dressed as lamb, it's O-K. As long as you highlight, texturise and keep away the frizz (I could go on, but I won't). But do not – I repeat, do NOT – wear your hair long and grey.
>
> Unbelievably it *is* possible to 'accentuate your femininity and embrace your years'. Seriously?
>
> And, lastly, because I'm not sure I can take any more: 'Just because you are over 40 doesn't mean you can't have a cute haircut.' This last, illustrated by a pixie crop on a 25-year-old Keira Knightley.

There are so many different pressures colliding here that I hardly know where to start. Embrace your greys! Embrace your age! Accentuate your femininity! Age is just a number! Don't give in to ageing! Age gracefully! Don't look your age! Look good for your age! Oh, and if you're going to 'embrace your grey', be sure you do it naturally. Lop it off when the clock strikes 40! Beware the frizz! (Have they heard of Grace Coddington, the formidable former creative director of US *Vogue*, she of the wonderful frizzy orange hair?) Layer on layer of judgement accompanies pretty much anything women do – especially when it's related to our appearance. We do it to ourselves (I pride myself on being my own greatest critic, especially where my appearance is concerned), and we do it to each other. I wonder whether, sometimes, just occasionally, we are guilty of judging other women, in part, to vindicate our own decisions. You only have to look at the vitriol that accompanies any debate around, say, motherhood or pregnancy to see that nine times out of ten women's most savage critics are other women who've chosen the opposite path.

When journalist Sali Hughes posted on Instagram that she was planning to go the whole hog and have her brunette shoulder-length hair stripped back and dyed silver/platinum/ whatever to get the whole grey thing over with in one go, she fell foul of exactly that. 'Both social acquaintances and women online I'd never met were horrified that I or anyone else would choose not to let nature take its course and apparently felt completely comfortable in telling me point blank to step away from the bleach,' she wrote in an article for The Pool soon after. 'While some women felt I'd look "too old", many others felt personally offended and let down by my decision, telling me repeatedly that I should "grow old gracefully", an expression more likely to send me hurtling down a path towards extreme facelifts and a cryogenic chamber.' A glance at her Instagram shows her hair is a deep glossy brunette. She looks bloody fabulous.

Anna Murphy was similarly dumbfounded by the reaction to her decision to go grey; her being fashion director of *The Times* it was even deemed worthy of an 'at once admiring and audibly bemused' mention on Radio Four. 'Suddenly my hair [was] not so much my thing, as a whole other thing,' she says, 'a separate entity, one that merits comment and discussion, that provokes bafflement in some ("What are you trying to prove?" asked one friend) and – to my surprise – admiration in others ("You are so brave. I wish I could do it," is a common response from women). Often the bafflement and the admiration seem intertwined.'

There's that word again: brave. It's one that comes up time and again. Elinor Carucci, author of the photographic book, *Midlife*, in which she documents her own journey through her forties and fifties and beyond, puts it like this: 'People say the work is brave and I take the compliment but I feel it's more like an attempt at connection.'

Helen, 45, was more no-BS about it. 'I stopped dyeing my hair last summer. Mostly I like it, sometimes not. Fuck it though! It's my hair! Mostly people have been kind, but I am tired of being told I'm brave. Brave is fighting cancer or rowing the Atlantic or Greta Thunberg. Accepting the natural colour of my hair is not brave!'

I get this. I heard it over and over when I posted a picture of my grey on Instagram. I was brave for considering going grey in the first place and even more so for posting a frankly not particularly attractive picture of myself with limited makeup first thing on a Tuesday morning. (Don't be fooled, I probably took 30 pictures before I settled on the first one because my forehead looked less wrinkled, plus I did fill in my non-existent eyebrows beforehand.) But it's not brave. If anything it's a bit insecure; it's as much saying, 'Look at my grey hair and tell me I'm doing the right thing' as saying, 'This is me, take it or leave it.'

Some applauded 'letting the grey shine' (when shiny is the last thing my grey is) and letting 'nature take its course', several who were trying to go grey said they were struggling: 'Sometimes I look in the mirror and ask myself why I'm doing this,' admitted @sarahcairncross, 'but mostly I'm loving the silvers and the self-acceptance. Some friends and family think I'm bonkers of course ...'

'I started going grey at 17. I've dyed it since then,' says @msmagpiespy, 44. 'Recently I grew the underneath out to see what it looked like, and I just didn't feel myself. I wanted to love it, but I've dyed it back and now I feel good again.'

'Personally I feel like I'm fading away when the grey comes in (I'm 45). I've spent most of my life playing small and not being seen, but I may yet get brave and don't want to fade just yet,' said @voiceovergirl. Ah, the old invisibility chestnut again. Wherever we go, whatever we do, we ultimately hit up against it. But I can't help wondering, in this case at least, whether going grey isn't actually the most visible option of all. Or one of them.

'It's the bloody pressure on females again,' commented hairdresser and book reviewer Nina Pottell. 'Being told to embrace their grey hair. If that's what someone wants to do then hooray and if they don't then hooray, too.'

It all boils back down to identity. The decision to go grey or pink or blonde or ginger is making a decision about who we are and who we want to be as we move forward into the next phase of our lives. Which is why it's often a decision we make when our life enters a period of flux. Fashion director and editor Anne-Marie Curtis took the decision to grow out her grey when she left her role as editor-in-chief of *Elle*. 'Since everything else was in transition, I thought, "Why not? New me, new hair, etc." It's taken ten months and I am a lot greyer now than I was then. Of course there are all kinds of analogies about how my "personal journey" the past year has been mirrored by that of my hair. A decision to change, the occasionally messy, confused and sometimes painful bit in the middle, then what do you know, you're there. Boom! I couldn't be happier with it.' And I'm not surprised; she looks like exactly the kind of soignée grey-haired woman of my dreams.

But not everyone ends up feeling as chic. 'I've always been dark-haired, but now I don't know what I am and I'm surprised by how much that affects me,' says @mcstrachan. 'I've stopped colouring over the last couple of years – I'm 44 now – and it's been fine. I love not being a slave to colouring appointments any more, but I can't in all honesty say I love being grey and I still get a shock when I see a photo.' For now she's decided to stick with it. For @msmagpiespy – who hasn't – the photos were a defining moment too: 'It was the before-and-after nature that photos will always take on that did it. I've always kind of looked the same, but gradually got older in my face. Body, hair colour, length much the same. Sudden change when I've never had that is scary. Like you say, who am I?'

American journalist Anne Kreamer went grey at 49. During research for her book about the process, *Going Gray,* she sent out pictures of the same person with grey hair and with dyed hair to hundreds of different people and asked them to guess their age. Typically, the people who received the grey picture would guess someone's age as only a year or two different from those who received the non-grey version. Perhaps the truth is, we don't look younger at all, we just look like a person who dyes their hair. After all, 75 per cent of US women now do so and the UK hair colour market is valued at £22 million.

It's not more feminist to dye your hair or not dye your hair. Nor is it feminist to criticise other women for doing it just because you wouldn't or vice versa. It's feminist to do what the hell you want with it as long as you feel great (and no children or animals were harmed in the process). It's feminist to let other women do the same. I have zero plans to cut off my hair because some dickhead on the internet thinks I look like a cat lady. Yep, I like cats. Yep, I've got long hair, what of it? And I'm not getting blonde highlights because some elements of the media decree blonde is the new purple. Frankly, I'd prefer purple. For me, the problem is not so much the grey as the 'going grey' and the texture ('those wiry little fuckers' as my friend Jo put it, peering critically at the crown of her head) and the nebulousness of my increasingly beige hair. For a while, if I caught sight of myself as I passed a shop window, all I saw was beige and a blob on the top of my neck where my hair and face used to be.

Having spent over 40 years with hair that was so definite, so loud, hair you could see across a crowded street and that entered the room before I did, I wasn't entirely sure I liked having hair that was so ... meek. Apologetic, even. It's not about whether I look old or young [or insert your age here], but whether I look intentional. Present. Decisive. Like I mean it. And whether, crucially, I look like me.

I recently had an epiphany following lunch with a friend at which I bemoaned the beige. 'Silvery red!' she objected. 'It's silver and red and blonde and people would pay a fortune to get that colour!' I dismissed her at the time, but the thought took hold. I could look at my nearly bum-length hair and see grey or I could look at it and see 'silver and red and blonde'. A silver vixen, if you will. And a colour that makes as much of a statement as my big red hair ever did.

'Fighting ageing is like the war on drugs. It's expensive, does more harm than good and has been proven to never end.'

Amy Poehler

6

A BRIEF RANT ABOUT ANTI-AGEING

One woman's love-hate affair with moisturiser

Anti-ageing *adjective*

Of or relating to any product or procedure claiming to reverse or slow down the effects of ageing. As in, anti-ageing beauty product. (*Collins English Dictionary* definition)

My definition: a way of making women feel lesser or afraid of getting older. Usually found in a bottle or a jar. *See also*, slow-age, pro-age, age-prevent, age-defy, anti-wrinkles, and all the other bollocks terms the beauty industry has come up with to avoid saying anti-ageing but still mean it. And usually modelled by women with no wrinkles at all or who have all their wrinkles airbrushed out.

I love moisturiser. I'm an addict. I have no off-button where skin-care is concerned. Makeup I can take or leave (except mascara) but I can't pass a skincare counter without buying something. Although, it's never one thing, is it? It's always part of a three for two, or a free gift if you buy, or I'll have the day and the night cream, and maybe I should throw in the eye cream. Oh, and there's serum, too. I couldn't tell you the last time I bought 'a' moisturiser. A single pot. All on its own. And the notion that I might wait for one thing to run out before buying a replacement ... how does that work? I get the concept when it comes to tomato ketchup and coffee and even antidepressants, but moisturiser? Only last Friday, I went into Boots to buy mouthwash and came out with three new vitamin C brightening products – day, night, eye (naturally) – despite the fact I have a big plastic box under the bathroom sink that's already full to overflowing with skincare products.

Here are some of the others I've bought in the last year or so: Beauty Pie Jeju AM/PM Moisture SuperInfusion, Triple Hyaluronic Acid, Uber Youth Serum and Super Retinol Night Renewal Moisturiser (in my defence, I had a membership I needed to use up!), The Ordinary Hyaluronic Acid and Natural Moisturising Factors + HA, Pestle & Mortar Renew Illuminating Lightweight Gel Cleanser, The Inkey List Caffeine Eye Cream, Origins GinZing (moisturising gel and eye cream), Boots No7 HydraLuminous Overnight Recovery Gel Cream ... See what I mean? Skincare is my vice. I can think of worse ones.

To a certain extent I blame having been what is laughingly called an 'industry insider'. While I am very much a punter not a pro where the beauty industry is concerned, several decades of being on the receiving end of free beauty products got me hooked on experimenting with new things. If I might once have had brand loyalty, that annihilated it, not to mention inuring me to the cost and embedding a skincare routine so central to who I am that once the freebies dried up, the box kept growing. Only my bank balance didn't.

But you know what I've realised I don't buy? Anti-ageing cream. Or, indeed, anything that uses the word 'age' to promote its alleged miracle-working prowess. Pro-age, slow-age, no-age. No ta. To double check, I went into the bathroom and looked through the crate again, and there's not a single one. For a moment, I feel quite proud of myself. But also a bit bemused, because it's not conscious. I'm not an anti-ageing activist (although I like the sound of it). I hadn't even noticed until now. But then I began observing myself, like an out-of-body secret shopper, and there it was. Online or in-store, I would swing straight past the products that promised to Benjamin-Button me the skin of a newborn by a week on Friday, drawn instead to the sciencey looking ones that make me feel in the know. If it majors on the ingredients (like The Inkey List, The Ordinary ...) and looks like it belongs in a French pharmacy or a pop-up in Hoxton, I'm sold. I'm no sucker for vegan or organic, or the dreaded 'clean beauty' (as opposed to dirty beauty?), but it turns out I do prefer brands that flatter my intelligence, that credit me with half a clue as to what the ingredients do. Or at least that make a token effort to appear to. The products that claim to solve a specific problem, like dull skin (currently I'm a bit obsessive about brightening, glowing and vitamin C) or highlight ingredients that are proven to 'work' (whatever *work* means to you). Who knew?

The truth is, I'm conflicted. Does the box of skincare under the bathroom sink somehow contradict my anti-ageing position just by existing? I mean, how can I complain about what it's called and yet still buy it – and consume it by the crateload – as long as it's called something else? Surely it doesn't matter as long as it does what it says on the jar?

But that's the point. It doesn't. It couldn't. Because age can't be wound back. Nor should it. We're all ageing, every single one of us. The lucky ones, at least. Only an idiot would literally be anti-ageing. So, the objection isn't to moisturiser – who doesn't want smoother, softer skin that doesn't flake to the touch? (I stopped using it for a few days just to see, and the result was dry, tight and a bit sore, red in patches – not pretty.) It's to having it sold to us (and by us I do mean women because I don't see it being sold to men the same way) in a way that makes us feel that simply by growing up, growing older, gaining experience, being a woman who's living life, we're doing something wrong. Sold to us in a way that makes us feel the contents of a jar is the only way we will ever be able to put ourselves right again.

I'm as gullible as the next person, my shopping habits are testament to that. Susceptible to minimalist packaging and a list of ego-flattering ingredients that would put Yotam Ottolenghi to shame. But it isn't just about the implausibility of the promise (we all know, in our hearts, that age can't be anti-ed, nor should it be), it's the covert insult that's hidden inside it: that younger is better, that older is wrong, that ageing as a woman is the worst thing you can do. Promising to turn back the clock in 28 days implies it needs to be turned back. The recently released MenoReverse, from Korres, implies that menopause can not only be reversed (bollocks to that) but that it's desirable to. That it will make your skin plumper, will make you somehow better, more youthful, fecund. (I love that word. Fecund.)

And don't toss me a token euphemism to make me feel better. It doesn't matter if it's defying it, slowing it or anti-ing it, if your product is focused on erasing those pesky signs of ageing, it's also focused on erasing me. I have lived a life to get here and I'm lucky I have. I have crow's feet. (I've had them ages, so long, in fact, that the first time I saw them reflected back at me in my sunglasses around the age of 30 I had no idea what they were. I just thought I'd scratched the lens.) But they're there. I don't love them. I don't hate them. I don't think about them. They're just me. I have freckles. Ditto. I have skin that now takes an hour every morning to lose the creases of the pillowcase I slept on. I have wrinkles where no wrinkles used to be. I use retinol at night under a bog-standard night cream, I use hyaluronic acid in the morning because it's a moisture magnet. Then I put a bog-stand-ard moisturiser on top. Sometimes I buy products that promise to give me back glow and products that promise to brighten my skin. Dull skin is, for me, the real downer of getting older. But it's not to reverse these 'signs of ageing', or even arrest them. It's to stop me looking like a paper bag by the time I'm 65.

Don't get me wrong, change is hard. To look in the mirror and see your face changing in front of you is harder still. Chin a little softer, eyebrows a little lower, under eyes a little baggier, frown a little darker. Thirty-three on the inside, 53 on the outside. But different things are hard for different women. While I was never 'a stunner' by society's standards, I am blessed with good skin and, so, I can live with those wrinkles – especially if I can temporarily magic back my glow. I buy mousses and creams and lotions and gels. I buy products that moisturise, products that rehydrate and products that claim to de-bag. But I don't have treatments. I have never had Botox or fillers or lasers or lifts. In a way, tweakment culture has made the decision easier for me. I simply don't like the photoshopped look. But plenty of people do, and, if you can afford it, it's really no big deal any more. Unless you're feeling the pressure because you won't get the job, or the roles, or the dates on Tinder. Then it's another story. But if you want to have tweakments, if they make you feel better or happier or just more relaxed at the end of a long hard week, then they might be for you. If your idea of heaven is to never know how you might have looked at 65, and you have the budget, then heaven is within your grasp. At some point, I may well look like your nan, but I prefer to think Charlotte Rampling

I'm not anti-ageing, I'm pro it. I just want to do it with slightly smoother, brighter skin. So don't patronise us, beauty companies. Don't shower us with euphemisms that mean the same thing and pretend you've listened and moved on. Put your money where your biggest untapped market is and listen to your customers instead.

Then, just as I was finishing this, two things happened:

Firstly, I was passing Boots and in the window I saw a picture of a mid-life woman – freckled, crow's feet, laughter lines, you name it. Even her chest was a bit crinkly. At first I just assumed she must be flogging Tena. But she wasn't! She was selling skin-care! And it wasn't even called anti-ageing! Miracles do happen. Hats off Boots No7, I salute you. BUT. (Why is there always a but?) Just as I was about to get complacent (and rewrite this chapter), the second thing happened. Novelist Kate Weinberg messaged me on Instagram: 'Walked past a beauty salon in London the other day and noticed they had this as a tagline: "Here ageing is optional!" Was so preposterous/sad I didn't know whether to laugh or cry!' she wrote.

Wow, talk about one step forwards, two steps back. I could be wrong but ageing ain't optional. Well, it is, but the other option ... it's not exactly preferable. So just in case you're still not clear, dear beauty industry, here's what women think about anti-ageing:

'Anything that claims to be anti-ageing is selling a myth.'
Deborah, 48

'Hate anti-ageing as a statement. Hate hate hate it!'
Helen, 45

'Once you've suffered loss or health scares, "anti-ageing", as a phrase, seems absurd. But that's something I've been tamed into. It mattered to me when I was younger. Now it doesn't. I do want to look the best 50 I can, but I no longer feel someone saying I look younger is a plus. I don't care. I'm here, some of my loved ones aren't.'
Karen, 50

'I loathe the whole anti-ageing thing. What's wrong with looking our age? Why is every line and wrinkle something to be fixed? There's a whole generation of women who will never know how they would have looked at 65. That's a loss.'
Fi, 51

'I have no great anti-ageing secrets (and slightly recoil from the term), but the two things I think are the most important as one gets older are a) looking after your teeth and b) exercise. There's not a face cream in the world worth putting on if you have receding gums.'
Nigella Lawson on turning 60 in The Sunday Times Style

'Our society has such a negative attitude to ageing. It's a privilege and an honour to have a long and happy life and I want to preserve and celebrate my skin and body as best I can at every stage and phase of my life. I love natural, clean skincare, a small touch of Botox and facial massage. I think you should approach ageing with peace and grace but do everything you can to help heal your skin. Being black and having oilier skin, ageing isn't such a large concern as I will probably look like this until I'm in my seventies, like my mum. She's 73 and looks amazing.'
Ateh Jewel, 42

'Dispassionately speaking, anti-ageing products make me sad: there's nothing wrong with ageing and even if there were it's not something that can be halted by products. BUT I'm suggestible. I'm affected by the messages that women should look young, slim and beautiful. And I get excited about 'magic' products. In my innermost heart I KNOW they won't make much difference while at the same time I'm willing to suspend disbelief. However, having said all that, I ENJOY skincare, I love the ritual of cleaning and moisturising, I love the feel of glidey products and when they smell nice, it gives me a real lift.'
Marian Keyes, 56

'I'm obsessed with skin creams and makeup and spend more now than any time in my youth.'
Paula, 49

'I really object to the glorification of youth and the idea that you have to have accomplished everything by the age of 30. "Older" women, skincare wise, are an under-served category and cosmetic firms are gradually waking up to this fact and their spending power.'
Rowena, 54

'There's a great deal to recommend, say, a face cream that smells nice, provides a smooth base for makeup, makes skin feel comfortable, moist and supple, look fresh and dewy and generally in great nick at any age. That is not an anti-ageing product, it's a great moisturiser and everyone should own one. An anti-ageing cream, however, sets its sights higher still; it also promises to slow the ageing process, to prevent the lines, discolouration and loss of volume that are entirely natural in all human faces as they get older. Anti-ageing skincare is controversial because it both implies that something is inherently wrong with looking one's age and at the same time promises to perform a feat that seems highly unlikely.'
Sali Hughes, Pretty Honest *(Fourth Estate)*

'I spend A LOT of money on skincare.'
Jojo Moyes, 50

'The term 'anti-ageing' has to be handled with care by the beauty industry. For some women, it's insulting and ageist ... Others couldn't care less what the product calls itself, as long as it delivers. There is, however, one thing all women have zero tolerance for, and that's being patronised. We don't tend to fall for ludicrous claims that wrinkles can be evaporated, and we know for a fact that the menopause can't be wished away ... Which is why brands tapping into insecurity and ignorance is unforgivable. Menopausal

women don't need quackery, they need evidence-based help for the things that are bothering them – along with a societal shift to view mid-life as something to be embraced. Change is happening slowly, but in the meantime, scaremongering brands will keep being called out. We might be menopausal, but we're not stupid.'
Saska Graville, founder of MPowered Women

'I hate the phrase anti-ageing or anything similar that's labelled with the word "age". Age doesn't matter, mindset and attitude do.'
Joanna, 52

'The anti-ageing messaging winds me up. I'll take getting older, as some of my friends have had this privilege denied to them.'
June, 46

'I don't have any mantras, I don't have any rules, I dress the way I please and I do what I please and I do everything for my own good.'

Iris Apfel

7

THE MENOPAUSE
OF CLOTHING

What to do when your clothes (and the fashion industry!)
turn against you, but you still want to look and feel like you

WTAF is age-appropriate dressing? Seriously. What is it, where
did it come from and who decides? It's a serious question. I
really want to know. Where do we get off age-shaming women
simply for what they wear? And I say we, because we all do it. I
spoke to more than 50 women about their relationship with
clothes and only 3 said they didn't do it to themselves on a regular basis. I did it to myself only this morning. I was thinking
about what to wear to write this chapter. Like playing the right
background music while you write, I really believe dressing like a
bag lady (which I often do, also a ten-year-old boy) has an
impact on your thought process. (I'm not saying it's science, it's
just a vibe.) I'm not talking about makeup, hair, the whole
shebang, I just mean that clothes can concentrate the mind.
Because getting dressed is making a decision about who you
want to be today, which is why getting dressed some days can be
such a massive ball-ache (sorry, vag-ache). And the person I
want to be today doesn't give a toss how old they are, would
happily throw the age-appropriate dressing brigade off a cliff,

and will take your so-called fashion rules and tell you where to shove them. And so, I write this wearing a Betty Boop T-shirt (Zara, yes, I know they're the Antichrist but it's a year old, and I love it) and comfy Isabel Marant joggers (ten years old and still going strong. Investment!).

I have spent a good part of the last few years of my life wrestling with my wardrobe. There are lots of things I can happily pin on the onset of menopause – you might have noticed – but, much as I'd like to, the breakdown of my style mojo that happened in my forties is not one of them. In fact, sharp intake of breath, I fear I have to go back a little further, and blame it on magazines. (No, this is not a skinny model conversation, I mean *editing* them.) But it was only when I hit perimenopause and almost simultaneously cut myself loose from the strictures of endless launches and dinners, presentations and twice-yearly fashion shows that I realised somewhere along the line my essence of Sam had gone AWOL. I hadn't noticed before, because I hadn't been looking – I had instead been doing my job. Dressing for the occasion. Dressing in armour. Dressing like a grown-up. Making like a fashion editor does, not like they say, i.e. developing a uniform and sticking to it regardless of what's on-trend, give or take a few tweaks.

So, when I left magazines, aged 46 going on 47 (what is it with the dread 47?) and the stays came off, I realised ten-year-old boy/ bag lady was all I had left. Not literally. I still had two wardrobes full of clothes. Expensive clothes. (Paid-for clothes. Albeit with press discount.) I had enough dresses to start a rental agency, if only I'd had the vision: cocktail dresses, work dresses, boho dresses, floral dresses, black dresses as far as the eye could see. LBDs, MBDs, GBDs (I'm making it up now). But ... I wasn't really a dress girl. Am not a dress girl. And haven't been since my early teens.

I was also not a heels girl, and yet I had an entire cupboard with shelves full of shoes: floor-to-ceiling Marni, Louboutin,

Prada, Jimmy Choo ... Strictly car-to-fashion-show shoes. The kind of shoes you can only really wear if you never walk anywhere. I had been dressing for the person I had to be at work. That person – well, that person's style – was not me. Admittedly I had an extensive collection of black trousers too, all with minuscule differences that made them 'worth the investment' – and wore them whenever I got the opportunity, with a black leather jacket (Theory, cost a fortune, cost per wear total bargain, still got it, still love it), three or four silk shirts on rotation and the dreaded heels (for when anyone could see my feet). So that, I guess, was my uniform. The real me, underneath the work me. But after I left magazines, every day I'd get up, stand in front of all those clothes (and all that money! Sob!) and wonder why I had nothing to wear for who I was now. Then I would put on the jeans (skinny, boyfriend or black-coated) that I'd left on the floor the night before, bung on a T-shirt and outsize shirt, Dr Martens or Converse, and go. (Like I said, a ten-year-old boy or a teenage Lemonheads fan, circa 1990s.)

The nadir came when, after the launch of The Pool, we won an award (called a Webby; it's a big deal in digital media). The Pool's co-founder Lauren Laverne and I went to New York to collect it. I had grabbed a black trouser suit out of the wardrobe from my editing days, and planned to team it with some stupid shoes and a vintage tee. When the agony got too much, I figured, I'd revert to Converse. I was proud of myself. I still had it. And I hadn't wasted any time or money worrying about it. I'd defaulted to uniform. Oh, the hubris.

It was only when I started getting ready that evening that I put on my suit for the first time and discovered the trousers didn't do up any more (now the spare tyre I definitely *can* blame on peri-menopause. And chocolate.). They weren't that old. They weren't a tight cut. They had always fitted perfectly, which is to say, slouchy. It hadn't occurred to me to check and I hadn't brought a spare outfit – smugly, I'd showed off about travelling light. For a fruitless 45 minutes I hurtled around SoHo, looking for another pair of trousers. But it was May, it was not a 'how to do black for summer' summer, and cool black trousers – or even uncool ones – were nowhere to be found. Not even in New York. So I spent the entire night with the button undone, pushing my food around my plate and praying the zip wouldn't unfasten; keeping my jacket on in spite of the heat to hide my spare tyre. Far from the cool start-up founder of my fantasies, I felt uncomfortable, hot, middle-aged and fat. I felt (and, I imagined, looked) like a gate-crasher in a room full of the great, the good and the young of digital media. (I shouldn't have worried because, like my nan always said, no one was looking at me. And they really, really weren't.) Added to which my bloody new shoes had started to pinch before we even reached the end of the block. My fail-safe go-to 'smart but cool' outfit had let me down. Three and a half thousand miles away from the rest of my clothes, the just-wear-black-and-add-a-glam-accessory strategy that had seen me through the previous decade or two had turned to shit. What was I going to do now?

The logical answer – the kind of answer a man might suggest (sorry to generalise, hashtag not all men, but it is) – is either buy a new suit or go on a diet. Possibly both. But logic doesn't really come into our emotional relationship with clothes, does it? When your clothes let you down like that, it's *personal*. 'We're not talking about a bit of fading here or a slight outdatedness there,' wrote Caitlin Moran in *The Times*. 'Instead your clothes suddenly and actively hate you. They want to destroy you, both physically and mentally. And this is something that happens, inevitably and unavoidably, to every woman over 40. In your mid-forties you have to put the "war" into your wardrobe.' And all over the land, thousands and thousands of fortysomething women nodded sadly as they black-bagged their favourite miniskirts and skinny jeans.

I hadn't known it, but I was on a wardrobe-identity tightrope. OK, so my clothes no longer fit. But that was secondary. The real question was *who* did I want them to fit anyway? With the whole notion of who I was in flux, how could I expect my clothes to morph effortlessly to the new me when I wasn't even halfway there myself?

Yes, my body had changed shape, the weight, as we've already discussed, had gone on quite literally overnight and what used to suit me, what used to pass for effortless ... well, my fail-safes were not fail-safe any more. Happily (sort of), the breakdown of my relationship with my personal style (with personal style getting custody of my previous body) coincided with the advent of athleisure, the stateless perimenopausal woman's best friend. Stretchy. Elasticated. But on-trend. It was win/win. I bought three pairs of Whistles 'office joggers' (not all at once, but in very quick succession) and for a couple of years wore nothing else except for boyfriend jeans, 99 per cent of the time with trainers and an M&S men's crew neck jumper. (They're good, I highly recommend them. In fact, I'm an advocate of requisitioning menswear in general.) I looked all right, I think. I didn't look too closely, if I looked at all. I didn't need to. I wore the same thing every day.

I was busy, I had found a 'uniform' that made me feel 'relevant' (i.e. not 'past it' in fashion speak) in a young working environment, and also in my life, but I wasn't happy. I love clothes. I love looking at them. I love filling a basket online and leaving them there overnight in the hope that someone will accidentally buy them for me. I even love buying them, when I can afford to. TBH I love that a bit too much. And I love looking at the way other women wear them. (I'm a total magpie for street style.) I love the way a great outfit can make you feel. And, like everyone else, I hate the way a bad one does. I have never, ever, loved trying them on, but who does? Suddenly all that was gone and I wasn't even 50.

What changes first, the body or the clothes, is anyone's guess.
So I made a project of it. I set out to work out what had gone
wrong and put it right. I did lose some weight – because I have
internalised patriarchal ideals of how women should look (i.e.
young and thin), and I felt better without my own personal life
buoy permanently around my middle. (Although that still comes
and goes.) But still, my go-to clothes and my go-to stores – the
ones where I knew that a size 12 actually was a size 12 – didn't fit,
not properly, not like they used to.

'When you get older, you're fucked because your body just isn't
a uniform shape,' says Kate Spicer, 50. 'You may remain a size 10,
or whatever, but your proportions are slightly different, and it's
not quite clear where you go in and where you go out, so cheap
clothes just don't really work any more.'

Brutal, but true. In the main, the fashion industry quite literally cuts its cloth for teenage bodies and doesn't acknowledge that
women of 40, 50, 60 and beyond still want to look in the mirror
and recognise themselves, even if it does take a bit more work –
and better-quality fabric – to pull it together. The fashion industry has no interest in expending its energy cutting clothes to fit
your thickening body, no matter how much money you've got.
(It's not called the male gaze for nothing. And the fashion industry is, like most industries, particularly the media, staffed largely
by women and run by men.) So caught up in image is the fashion
industry that even brands who make amazing well-made, well-
priced clothes for women of all ages, brands whose main
customer group is women over 40, are reluctant to shout about it,
certainly don't see them as their target audience and thus won't
market to them. (There are, of course, notable exceptions, like
Universal Standard in the States, and Australian lingerie brand
Lonely, whose diverse model choices stand out in a haze of young,
white, thin faces.)

'They still target 25- to 30-year-olds even though everyone
knows they have little money,' one fashion insider told me,

naming a brand owned by a large Scandinavian high-street retailer, which has shops all over the UK. I've shopped there and, if you live in a major city, I'm pretty sure you have too. 'Their biggest customer age group is 40+, but you wouldn't know it from their imagery ... they think that by targeting 40-plus they will put off younger customers. I can't think of a brand that shows cool 40-plus women wearing cool clothes that we would want to wear ...'

'We do not have to dress a certain way because we are a certain age,' concurs fashion blogger and stylist Alyson Walsh (aka That's Not My Age), in a blog written to coincide with her 56th birthday. 'With my casually glamorous clothes, flat run-around shoes and natural grey-ish hair, I look completely different to the way my mum looked in her fifties. Ageing today is bound up with mindset, lifestyle and self-expression.'

'I feel like my mum, now 70, has spent her whole adult life not being able to find clothes she likes, so this is not a new phenomenon,' says Helen, 45, 'despite the fact that what my mum wanted to wear at 45 would be very different to what I wear (fashions notwithstanding). It's age-old. Once a woman is past her thirties, the fashion and beauty industries have no interest in us.'

Instead, what we end up with, if we're lucky, is the catch-all 'older women' often used to apply to all women over 40 (40!). I mean, I'm 53, my mum is 75, my stepson's wife is 40. We have different lives, different styles, different bodies and different budgets, but we all want affordable, stylish, well-cut clothes that make us feel like us.

Leisurewear is no better. Shelley Silas, 61, has been running for the last five years. 'I love my kit,' she admits. 'I have a chest of drawers dedicated to my running gear and a rack for my trainers. There are many other women like me, but we are never represented. At a Stonewall Fundraiser a few years ago, I happened to sit beside a man who was head of diversity for Adidas in Germany

(I love Adidas). When I asked why there were no mature women on their posters or online, he said (and he was very sensitive), "You're not our market, you're not the person we aim for." I pointed out that the older generation is generally the one with the money. "Yes," he said, "but if there was a pair of celebrity trainers that cost £300, would you buy a pair?" I said no, of course not. "There you go," he said. Basically he was saying that we are not fashionable. I totally disagree. Obviously I wouldn't spend £300 on a pair of bloody trainers ... I spent £90 on mine ... but that's hardly cheap!'

Which brings me to representation. There is a growing trend towards using older models in fashion and beauty campaigns, but trend is what it is. Celine used Joan Didion (aka one of the coolest women in the world, who happens to be 85 and bird-thin) to sell sunglasses a few years ago, Saint Laurent used Joni Mitchell, and Calvin Klein used Lauren Hutton. There are so-called 'senior influencers' who are also making a name for themselves (Baddiewinkle, Iris Apfel), but there's a tendency towards the very quirky, the very old, and the very thin. And white. They are used to make a statement, not for identification; a fling that usually lasts a season at most, before the diversity baton is passed on to race or body positivity. Box ticked, job done and it's back to business as usual. It's not a shift towards a new normal, it's a publicity stunt. Where are the women in the middle? The women like us? One grey-haired 70-year-old model might tick the age box, but it is in no way a step change; after all, there are as many different ways of being over 40 as there are women.

The only truly legit one I can think of is the American model and musician Leslie Winer, now 61. Big in the eighties, she returned to modelling as the face of Vivienne Westwood's Spring/Summer 2014 campaign, in her early fifties. Amber Valetta, 44, and Laura Bailey, 47, make the occasional reappearance, but I can't think of many more.

'Less than 2 per cent of advertisers feature Gen X and Baby Boomers,' says Debra Hepburn, 58, who founded Young British Designers ten years ago to celebrate young British talent and encourage consumers to shop original. 'When a catwalk or an editorial or a well-known fashion house features an older woman there is a massive noise made and huge (commercially viable) applause is created. But this should be the norm. That all women, of all ages, life stages and appearances, appear, without a fanfare, across all of our media.'

Fifty-six per cent of Generation X women feel ignored by the high street. When you ask all women over 45, that increases to 70 per cent. Is it any wonder that, according to a report by the International Longevity Centre UK, the fashion industry stands to cost itself as much as £11 billion in the next 20 years if it continues on this blinkered trajectory?[13] But more than that, in what world is that OK? In what world does a business predicated on profit ignore a potentially huge market because it doesn't much like the look of their faces (and bodies)? In what world does that market put up with it?

'It really annoys me,' says Deborah Campbell, 49, founder of Deborah Campbell Atelier, who has worked in the fashion industry for over 20 years. 'I'm tired of the structure of the fashion industry that still feels it's relevant to dictate that age is a way of storytelling and selling product. Brands should use a variety of women who represent that group. Millennials will not put up with this if brands don't change.'

She's not kidding. In fact, there are plenty of things about being north of 50 that I'm pretty sure millennials will not put up with. But why should we wait for them to turn up? I can just imagine the CYW I used to work with turning 47 and watching their Facebook feeds blow up with tent dresses. (And no, it's nothing to do with your search history. It's as basic as they know your birthday and have taken it upon themselves to decide you're no longer allowed to buy certain things.)

As we perspire our way through the perimenopausal identity maze, we could be mistaken for feeling like the fashion industry is wilfully trolling us, as if bombarding us with what a friend on Facebook called 'basically burkhas' will send us into hiding where it clearly thinks we belong. Which brings me to The Fashion Rules. Let's play the Google game again. (I'm not going to do this every chapter, promise, but this one is special.) Google 'style rules': you'll get 1.7 billion hits. 'Fashion rules': 1.4 billion. 'Age appropriate': 2.2 billion. 'Dress your age': 2.7 billion, and watch your laptop explode. I do this exercise only to illustrate that laying down rules about what we should and shouldn't wear – and shaming those who refuse to abide by them – is big business. It's underpinned the fashion industry since it was invented. Young is cool and old is not. Coco Chanel created rules we're still adhering to now – although at least plenty of those (straps on handbags, pockets, trousers for women) are female friendly.

'I'm not sure when I first became aware of The Fashion Rules,' says Debra Hepburn. 'That certain shapes, colours, lengths, cuts didn't suit certain body types and apparently, hugely importantly, certain ages. That "helpful" but repressive narrative seeped into my consciousness via the fashion press, my mum ("are you really going out like that?"), my colleagues at work ("ooh, that's unusual, I couldn't wear that/you're very brave" [there it is again]) and, of course, relatively recently, social media. I became more and more aware of it the older I got.'

Debra's awareness of the rules really came crashing in after she launched YBD. 'I was too curvy, too old, not tall enough, not on-trend enough. I wore our brilliant designers' clothes, shoes, accessories because I loved them. But I hid away in case I embarrassed them by not being a young, tall and beautiful size 8 or less.' Then, in 2016 she got 'brave' and put a picture of herself on YBD's Instagram. 'I did it because I was wearing the most gorgeous hand-block-printed skirt by one of our designers and I wanted to share how wonderful it was and how it made me feel wearing it. The response blew me away. I received a deluge of DMs all asking me to wear more, share more. And the skirt sold out. And the designer was not embarrassed to see old, curvy me, wearing her creations. Far from it. She was delighted. Seems most designers get an absolute rush from seeing real people wearing their designs and loving them in real life. Who knew?'

Since then, Debra has begun posting more pictures of herself. 'I always hesitate and think: really, does anyone truly want to see this old bag talking about what she wears and why she cares about it? But then I get all the responses from women telling me I've encouraged them to "stop dressing their age", that I've kicked them "up the arse and out of a rut", that I've inspired them to start enjoying fashion again.'

This reaction also prompted Debra to start advising customers, 'often professionals at the top of their career games, almost exclusively women aged over 40', to take another look at clothes they thought they 'couldn't' wear. Their responses were eye-opening:

'Oh, I can't wear pink because I have red hair.'
'I have to wear a high neckline as my chest is all wrinkly.'
'My husband says I have a short waist so I can't wear anything fitted.'
'But I'm 50 now, I can't wear a skirt that ends above the knee!'
'I have huge feet [size 40, the UK average] so I need to wear dark shoes.'
'I'm hot all of the time so can't wear sleeves but I can't go sleeveless as it'll show my bingo wings.'

'They were endless. They are still endless. These are beautiful older women tying themselves in knots about what they're allowed to wear (or not),' Debra added.

117

Joanna Davies, 52, of Black White Denim, tells the same story. 'The biggest battle we have as strong, independent women in middle age is that we have been socialised to start giving up and slowing down at 50ish when, in fact, we are doing anything but,' she says. The following are all heard daily in her fitting rooms:

'I'm too old for that.'
'My daughter would say I looked like mutton dressed as lamb.'
'My husband doesn't like blah, blah or blah.'
'I'm 53, I can't get away with that.'
'I would have worn that back in the day.'
'My kids would laugh at me.'
'I need to tuck my muffin top in.'
'I can't show the top of my arms.'
'I've put on so much weight.'
'Can you see my back fat?'

'The list is truly endless,' says Jo. 'My job is to give women of our age permission to refocus on what they WANT to wear and WANT to look like and not what the rest of the world is telling us we "should" do.'

Controlling the way women dress is in no way a new thing. 'What we have to remember is that clothes for women – as every other part of the female existence – have always been circum-scribed by a huge amount of rules and regulations about what is and is not appropriate,' Anna Murphy, fashion director of *The Times* and author of *How Not to Wear Black*, tells me. 'Putting age to one side, it's easy to forget how comparatively recently, for example, it was not OK for women to wear trousers. The Second World War was the first time women wore trousers *en masse* and newspapers actually had front-page headlines saying "Will slacks turn our women slack?!" Like everything else, it's just another way of policing women.'

In the meantime, if we're not age-shaming ourselves, leave it to the media to do it for us. They've been doing it for decades, after all. The examples are legion but my favourite is model Helena Christensen, 50, daring to leave the house in a bustier. She wasn't going to buy a pint of milk (and who cares if she was?), she was going to fellow model Gigi Hadid's birthday party. She looked amazing. Not that that's relevant. A day or so later, the former editor of British *Vogue*, Alexandra Shulman, wrote this: 'We might like to think that 70 is the new 40 and 50 is the new 30, but our clothes know the true story.' She went on to say that it was 'disturbing and slightly tragic' for a woman of Helena's great age to flaunt her body. I mean, FFS. Is it any wonder we're scared to wear what we bloody well want to, even if we *can* find it?

Which, we mainly can't. The litany of complaints is endless. Here are just a few from the women I spoke to:

Julie, 56: 'I have put on a fair amount of weight over the last few years, which is partly down to menopause and partly due to life happening. And now I'm faced with blah clothes that fit rather than look good. Where are the retailers who offer larger sizes in their normal range? Next, M&S and Monsoon seem to be the only high-street (read "affordable") ranges who offer above a 16, but their clothes are uninspiring and dull. Is there anyone who offers clothes that are a bit different, a bit edgy? Does anyone cater for people who were teenagers in the seventies and eighties? I don't think so. I funk it up as much as I can, but it's so demotivating.'

Juliet, 50: 'I fell out of love with my clothes last summer. All the fail-safe shift dresses that I wear to work seemed to actively hate me. I still don't love my clothes but have started buying well-cut things and adding elements of colour. I've never returned so many clothes in my life as I do now. I don't even know what looks nice any more.'

Lisa, 52: 'I don't know what I'm supposed to be dressed like. I'm worried I'll look ridiculous in Top Shop and ASOS, yet I'm not feeling Hobbs, Jigsaw, Laura Ashley. I'm in limbo. I'll be dead before I'm in a polo shirt and fleece!'

Paula, 49: 'I'm more picky where I shop and definitely have found that you need to pay more as you age – basically you need a better cut, better fabric (no flimsy rubbish), sharp tailoring, which you don't get with ASOS, etc. I can't stand sites where there is tons of choice. It's so painful. I've come to despise fast fashion. It does make me mad that most brands don't market to our age group properly. I love that brands like Rixo add a grey-haired model and have them next to the young skinny girl. We have the disposable income and the loyalty they need to court but brands still don't get it.'

Everyone agreed the fashion industry was missing a trick ignoring women over 40 – and that includes women who work in it. Jane Shepherdson, one of the most stylish women in fashion, who has influenced more of our wardrobes than most during her days leading Top Shop and then Whistles, says her look hasn't changed for more than 30 years. 'My current style is a structural shirt/blouse – Isabel Marant, Arket, Cos – worn with jeans from Acne, which I've bought for ages ... or if I'm short of money, Uniqlo fit well, too. My Dr Marten monkey boots I bought in 2017 are still going strong and my new Veja trainers are great.'

She concedes, however, that knowing your style is key. Having her encyclopaedic brand knowledge helps too! For the other 99 per cent of the population, what the hell do we do? 'I do think it's more difficult for women who are less confident, as the imagery that all the brands use is usually of a woman around 25/30 years old, so it's hard for them to get an idea of what's age-appropriate,' she says. 'Then again I have a BIG problem with age-appropriateness – wear what you want at any age!' (Anna Murphy agrees: 'What's important is that what's on your rails should match your state of mind, not the number on your birth certificate,' she says.)

Now CEO of My Wardrobe HQ, Jane has unsurprisingly become a 'rental zealot'. 'I simply refuse to pay a huge amount of money for occasion dresses, or something for a wedding. I am a huge advocate of rental for those occasions, for a couple of reasons: firstly because there's a real Cinderella moment, wearing something that you could never afford to buy – it makes you feel fabulous. And secondly for the obvious sustainability reasons – it's not going to sit in the wardrobe and end up in landfill.'

Rental, vintage, sewing your own. In the face of sod-all interest from the fashion industry, we are increasingly turning to new ways to find clothes that don't patronise us. There's also, as Jane points out, an ever-growing sustainability issue that fashion in general, and the fast-fashion end of the high street in particular, is failing to address.

Helen, 45, puts her comparative contentedness down to the fact she makes her own clothes. 'I sew most of my own clothes, which means I can make what I want, within the limitations of my skill and time and what patterns are out there. (In the sewing world, thin, young, white and privileged still rule in terms of marketing and what sizes patterns go up to, but there has been a backlash and a lot of pattern companies have responded.) But if I want to make something cropped but a bit longer, I can do that. If I want sleeves or hemlines longer or shorter, if I want to add bloody pockets, I can do that. Most fundamentally, it means (again within my skill level) that I have clothes that fit me! I don't have my ideal wardrobe but I can wear the aesthetic I choose in the fabrics I want. It's not cheaper than fast fashion, but I can make a coat or a dress far cheaper than one from Whistles.'

Deborah Campbell stopped shopping altogether for a year and highly recommends it. 'I did this in 2012 and it really did change my habits,' she says. 'Buy less, choose well and shop my wardrobe is the way I live.' While the fans of vintage are queuing up to rave about it. 'I've always bought loads of second-hand stuff. But the boom in designer second-hand has totally revitalised my wardrobe in mid-life,' says Kate Spicer. 'Sites like Vestiaire and Hardly Ever Worn It. You don't have to fight in the changing room. You don't have to fight with the fact that the lovely thing you're looking at costs £2,000. I bought a Saint Laurent tweed blazer for £300 on Hardly Ever Worn It that I could never have afforded in the shop. It's an amazing jacket. I love it so much and I feel like that's what I should be wearing at my age: £1,500 blazers!'

'I am fortunate that I have always had the right figure for vintage clothes (I am 5 foot 3, size 10 to 12, with a very small high waist, narrow shoulders and rounded hips and a 32 DD bust) and most modern clothes are cut completely wrong for me,' says Carrie Cornell, 57. 'As my body changed, through pregnancy, childbirth and menopause, I haven't felt that I have "lost" my defining look, I've just adapted, found other influences, like TV (*The Crown, Fleabag, Killing Eve*) and discovered Instagram accounts like @enbrogue and @notbuyingnew. Style, fashion, craftsmanship, colours, patterns, textures, all make me happy.'

Anna Murphy is another colour champion. 'I've always loved clothes, I've always loved colour. I used to wear one or two bits of colour and keep the rest dialled down, but now I wear head-to-toe colour and pattern, and the way people react to me has completely changed. I'm 48 years old, and young men, for example, regularly come up to me because of my [grey] hair, because of what I'm wearing – not to hit on me, just to say how fabulous I look. I think that's because I'm dressing to express myself, to enjoy myself. It's not about following stupid trends and wearing trouser shapes that don't fit you and worrying about what you should be wearing when you're 50 not 30. It's about dressing in a way that truly embodies you and empowers you and that's an amazing thing. Fashion is a female superpower if you embrace it in the right way.'

Develop a new uniform, quality not quantity, buy less buy better, all come up again and again. Buy vintage, rent, edit out all the crap, follow smart women whose style you love on Instagram, regardless of their age and yours. Don't dress for anyone but you. Buy a full-length mirror, and get to know yourself in it. Compliment each other. If you see a woman you think looks fab, tell her so and make her day. (And take the compliment if you're on the receiving end ...) And, above all, if you love it, wear it, whatever you think anyone else might say.

And don't worry about brands. As Anna Murphy puts it, it's not where you buy, it's what you buy that counts.

I'm feeling optimistic, because I think there is another thing that has changed: our willingness to put up with the scraps the fashion industry can be arsed to toss us. As our bodies change, so does our attitude and with it our identity evolves. Like being 15, but with all the assets and experience of being 50 and fully sick of it.

'At 54 I came full circle back to where I started as a young, fashion-loving girl,' says Debra Hepburn. 'Just as the confidence of youth, of sheer unadulterated joy in fashion, unknowingly gave me my risk-taking attitude back then, there's a whole new dynamic now. We can choose to become recessive, invisible, irrelevant (and God knows hormone-driven days feel that way). Or we can celebrate our new-found fashion freedom. After all, we're no longer (I hope!) competing for the male gaze.'

'You get more yourself every time I see you,' a friend told me when I met her for coffee the other day. We were both wearing black skinny jeans, chunky boots, different colour T-shirts. Statement jackets. Lots and lots of layers! The same was true of her. I looked at her and saw a woman in charge of her life, comfortable in herself, at the top of her game. Not dressing to impress anyone but herself. So this morning, I looked in the mirror and I didn't see my thighs, or my stomach, or my chins. I saw me. Then I dressed for myself. I put on my Betty Boop T-shirt, my Dr Martens and my comfy joggers, and before I sat down to write I took a selfie. Happy that, after a long time AWOL, the woman in the mirror looked like me.

'When you come to age, if you have this broad identity [as being about your looks], what does it mean to get wrinkles and get closer to menopause? ... What happens to your identity as a woman if you're not fuckable and beautiful?'

Gwyneth Paltrow

8

AN END TO FUCKABILITY

Redefining 'sexy' when you no longer
fit society's bill of what's hot

'Would you wear shoes if you didn't have feet?'

We were halfway across the bridge that linked the two sites of my comprehensive school. Classes F3 and F4 moving like an amoebic blob from science on the 'girls' side' to English on the 'boys' side'. Grey concrete spanning a busy road, its waist-height rails a death trap waiting to happen. School gossip had it that the previous year a fifth-year girl was thrown off, into oncoming cars, as punishment for snogging another girl's boyfriend. She didn't die, but she did spend most of the term in hospital. That didn't stop the chaos of 11- and 12-year-old boys pushing, shoving and taking aim with muddy Adidas holdalls, girls clustering, shrieking, gales of mildly unconvincing laughter. The bridge was never a good place to be waylaid. It was to be scuttled across, and pray no one noticed you.

'Oi! Duracell!'

Uh-oh. I peered up through my fringe, confused. Was Robert Flanagan talking to me? I hoped not. Boys never bothered with me. Unless ... 'I said, would you wear shoes if you didn't have feet?' he repeated, his voice a jeer.

It was a trick question. I knew that from the silence that had fallen around us, drawing curious glances from older kids going in the opposite direction. Like hyenas, waiting to pick over the bones of someone else's prey.

There had to be a right and a wrong answer. But which was which? 'Erm ... no?' I guessed.

Wrong.

'Why d'you wear a bra then?' he yelled. And laughter exploded around me.

I was proud of my bra. I'd only just got it. Pale pink, 30 AA, from M&S (as pretty much everything was then). And what really stung was the truth of his jibe. I didn't need a bra. I didn't have any boobs, just bumps. But I was the only girl in the class who didn't wear one and, even though I had the 'excuse' of being one of the youngest in the year, wearing a vest had eventually become too much to bear. After months of asking, begging, cajoling, pleading, I'd finally bored my mum into buying me one. And now this. Hard evidence that however much I went through the motions, the popular girls would never let me into their bra-wearing gang, and the popular boys (and the unpopular ones, too) would never do anything but take the piss out of me. They would certainly never fancy me. And somehow, since moving from primary to secondary school, that had begun to matter. Too ginger, too blocky, too flat-chested, too good in class, too bad at sport. Too unpopular.

It took me woefully long to realise the safest way to survive was to pretend I didn't care. Instead, I adopted all the trappings of girldom: bra, makeup (smuggled out of the house in the morning, applied in the loos before first bell), hair, heels, skirt rolled up at the waist, and tried to make like I belonged.

I can't honestly say fuckability was something I gave a huge amount of thought to before Amy Schumer performed her sketch 'Last Fuckable Day'. But I knew, right then, on that day in 1977, that there was some intangible thing that girls who were liked by boys had – and I didn't have it. I mean, you only have to be asked so many times if you'd wear shoes if you didn't have feet by the class comedian to get the message that if you are a girl, you will be measured and found wanting – by society, by other girls, by boys. You may not be entirely clear what it is they are judging you on, but you do know that whatever it is you haven't got it.

Let's face it, fuckable wasn't even a thing till 'Last Fuckable Day' went viral in 2015. But Schumer didn't create fuckability, she just gave voice to something we always knew was there. That's why a five-minute comedy routine that could have just been an in-joke (admittedly between half the population) went from a late-night slot on Comedy Central to becoming part of the vernacular of the Western world. It's because there's scarcely a woman alive who didn't identify and snort herself silly over it. Even those who never really thought about whether or not they were fuckable before – or if they had, wouldn't have felt they fit society's definition of it, or cared less.

If you didn't see it, I advise you to run like the wind to YouTube and search 'Last Fuckable Day'. Or maybe F*ckable. They're peculiarly puritanical for a site where you can find a six-year-old accidentally watching Peppa Pig porn even with the filters in place.

Here it is, in a nutshell: out for a run one day, Amy Schumer stumbles across Patricia Arquette, Tina Fey and Julia Louis-Dreyfus having a boozy picnic lunch. As they down champagne and chug a litre of melted Ben & Jerry's they tell Schumer they're celebrating Dreyfus' Last Fuckable Day and proceed to initiate her in what it means to no longer be considered fuckable in Hollywood.

'In every actress's life you reach the point where the media decides you're not believably fuckable any more,' Dreyfus explains. 'Nobody overtly tells you,' Fey goes on, 'but there are signs. You know how Sally Field was Tom Hanks's love interest in *Punchline* and then 20 minutes later she was his mom in *Forrest Gump*?'

There are other signs: being cast in roles where you get to compete with 20-year-olds to shag 80-year-old men, the wardrobe department kitting you out in shrouds, movie posters that feature the interior of your house rather than the exterior of your body. Your best movies being remade with younger actresses ...

By these standards, they explain, Dreyfus has done well: allowed to stay fuckable all the way through her forties and into her fifties. Some mistake surely.

It's funny because it's true. And the funniest bit of all? When Schumer asks who tells men when their Last Fuckable Day is. After the others finally pick themselves up off the grass, Fey says patronisingly, because, really, what a dumb question: 'Honey, men don't have that day. They're fuckable for ever. They could be a hundred with nothing but white spiders coming out but they're fuckable.'

Bless their cotton socks, it doesn't occur to them we might not even want to fuck them any more. And why would it? In Hollywood, as in life, men have been writing the rules for centuries. And according to their rules, they don't have to look 20 – or even 40 – to get a 20-year-old girlfriend. Out in the real world, it's not much better. Men of 50 are called silver foxes, being made CEO and swiping left on women more than a decade younger than them. Harriet, 48 and recently separated from her husband of 24 years, decided she wanted to stick to men in her own age bracket (45–54) when she tried online dating. 'Under the question "do you want kids?" most of them were saying, "Yes, I think so, in the future." So it seems obvious that they don't want a woman of their own age because for me that's an option for one more year, at most.'

Sasha, 45, had a similar experience on the *Guardian* Souldestroyer (I mean, Soulmates) dating site four or five years ago, when she went on a date with a man ten years her senior. 'He told me I was "perfectly nice",' she laughs. 'But his "upper age limit" was 35.' She can 'see the funny side now but at the time it was bloody depressing'.

And, really, why wouldn't your average bloke in the street think they're entitled to behave like that when you have men like French author Yann Moix saying that 50-year-old women are 'too old' to love. 'The body of woman of a 50 is not extraordinary at all,' announces this clearly exceptionally hot 52-year-old.[14]

You can see where the problem lies. While men of 50 are hanging out on dating apps idly judging the fuckability of women 10 or 20 years their junior, women turn 45, 50, 55, if we're really lucky, and are suddenly only good for knitting, cooking, babysitting, and reminding the rest of their family whose birthday they've just missed ... Or, in Julia Louis-Dreyfus's case, getting clothes out of the dryer.

Until that point, Schumer's sketch is basically flawless, the template for all menopause celebrations to be held hereafter. A lesson in how to stick one to the patriarchy and redefine fuckability for yourself. So you'd think they'd have had actresses biting off their hands to star in it. But according to the team behind it, far from it. When it came to casting, the sketch was written with Susan Sarandon in mind ('Because she's had to carry the mantle of being the fuckable older actress for so long,' executive producer Jessi Klein told *Vanity Fair*[15], with Sigourney Weaver or Julianne Moore also on the wishlist. Not a chance. Apparently actresses for whom unfuckability was a little too close for comfort were slightly less keen to play along. (Or, perhaps more likely, their agents were ...) Hardly surprising in Hollywood where the Gods of Fuckability still reign.

But let's face it, fuckability, is not exactly new. Nor is it exclusive to Hollywood. Recently *Friends* star Lisa Kudrow said that back in the nineties a guest star told her he'd had no idea she was fuckable until she came out of hair and makeup ... (Bet you a tenner that was Charlie Sheen.) As far back as 1982, actress Debra Winger (then 27) was told by producer Don Simpson she wasn't fuckable enough to be cast in *An Officer and A*

Gentleman opposite Richard Gere. The movie, starring Winger and Gere, went on to be box office legend. Shows what he knew. Hollywood is just life writ larger and, though I wish they wouldn't, I'm not surprised women whose birthdays start with a five or a six are reluctant to draw attention to it just in case whoever keeps the unfuckable list realises they've missed their name off it.

But things are changing. Aren't they??? We live in an era of Weinstein and #MeToo, #TimesUp and #BelieveWomen. Surely the cult of fuckability is destined for the scrap heap? But when *Hollywood Reporter* recently ran a piece about menopause on screen, the reporter, Monica Corcoran Harel, found that 'more than 20 actresses in mid-life declined to be interviewed for this report'[17]. (Again that may well be their reps, not the actresses themselves.) It's not that different behind the camera. A friend of mine who was recently taken on by an LA-based script agent just short of her 50th birthday begged me to give her age as 49 when I interviewed her. Apparently he loved her work, but having an age that began with a five would have been a deal-breaker for him. The message: have an agent or a birthday but (if you're a woman) you can't have both.

But still! Let's be positive! I mean, there's Gwyneth Paltrow – admittedly no longer an actress but a 'wellness mogul' – speaking out about how 'menopause gets a bad rap and needs a rebranding'. She's right. (I don't doubt she's already got her eye on the commercial opportunity.) And then there are a whole host of actresses in their forties and fifties who – unlike the generation before them, which seemed to be modelled on the principle of 'we've got one (Meryl, Judi), we don't need another' – are not going anywhere. Actresses like Laura Dern, Reese Witherspoon, Viola Davis, Nicole Kidman, Sandra Oh, Helena Bonham Carter, Taraji P. Henson, Julianne Moore, Patricia Arquette ... (I could go on) whose careers are on fire. If anything, they're getting bigger than ever, and so are their mouths. (Patricia Arquette in particular has a nice sideline in Golden Globes speeches that bring the house down.) They're getting more outspoken, and with it, they seem to be getting more parts. And when they aren't, they're creating them for themselves. And the best thing of all? What I don't see, when I look at them, is fuckability. Beautiful, yes. Talented, yes. Sexy, yep. Extremely well maintained, for sure. Fuckable ... not so much.

I sent the Amy Schumer sketch to my menopause coven. 'I'm not sure how much fuckability has to do with purely age?' Rowena wrote back. She's right. Being fuckable means something darker, something more misogynistic than just being deemed sexually desirable ... It's not just desirable, it's pliable. It's not just young, it's young and hot. It's unthreatening. It's ultimately utterly lacking in agency. You're not there to act, you are there to be acted upon. Remember that scene in *Notting Hill* where a group of men on a nearby table say of Julia Roberts' character, Anna Scott: 'She's absolutely gagging for it.' And then continue, 'Do you know that in over 50 per cent of languages the word for "actress" is the same as the word for "prostitute"? And *Anna* is your definitive *actress*.' It's that. It's Harvey Weinstein picking off young, talented, new-to-LA actresses one by one. It's news producers wielding their power to take what isn't theirs from young, ambitious women who've been trained to believe that it's not within their rights to say no, and enforce it. And I'm 100 per cent certain it's not what anyone goes into acting, or any other career, for.

Fuckability has had many guises over the decades. But it all boils down to power and not having any. Because fuckable is more insidious; it implies some sort of ownership over you and your body. Fuckable says you *would*. Fuckable implies you'd let them. The audience, the internet trolls, the teenage boys in their bedroom, brought up on the-geek-will-get-the-girl fantasies, the entitled middle-aged men who still (for now) run the show. They *could*. It's the hotness ratings on dating apps. It's the rape threat pile-on on social media. Things that are never, ever aimed at men.

I grew up in the dark ages that were the seventies when, as we're now discovering, it seemed to be a given that men could do whatever the hell they wanted and women understood that they just had to put up with it. Stuart Hall was on primetime, Jimmy Saville could fix it and Benny Hill was still on TV, literally dressing as a perv and chasing a 'bevy' of barely clad 'lovelies' around the screen for 30 minutes. (That was it. That was the gag.) Even as a small child I understood that his 'angels' were whatever that decade's version of fuckable was and not thinking it was hysterically funny made you, well, a bit odd. (Humourless feminist in training.) Most of the time I was more preoccupied with how I could get to live in Laura Ingalls Wilder's Little House on the Prairie or Anne Shirley's Green Gables. That and the fact I was never going to get a Girl's World for Christmas. But subliminally, I already knew I didn't fit the mould. I would never be an 'angel'. And even Girl's World didn't come with ginger hair.

The closest thing I can think of to fuckability before fuckability was invented is man-pleasing. Doing the right thing, saying the right thing, looking the right way. I was never very good at it and anyone who valued it rarely gave me more than a passing glance. The only time one did, it ended in the hotel room at the start of Chapter 2. What happened may not have turned me into a man-pleaser but it gave me a people-pleasing habit it took three decades (and, coincidentally or not, the advent of menopause) to break.

Being a young woman in the 21st century hasn't changed much in that regard: your place in the popularity scale is assigned to you based on youth and beauty, yes, but also your willingness and ability to fit in. (Oestrogen isn't sometimes called the biddability hormone for no reason.) The difference is, the internet is now full of young people pushing the boundaries of what defines us. But for every Slumflower telling you How To Get Over A Boy, or Laura Bates calling out the micro and macro aggressions of the

Everyday Sexism that were part and parcel of my youth (and most of my adulthood too), or Florence Givens reminding us we don't owe anyone pretty, there's a whole other community tweaking and facetuning and filtering their way to fuckability. Because if there's one thing the tweakment face says it's I'm fuckable.

Still, maybe the days of learning early and learning hard that you don't fit the bill are numbered. (Although I watch my god-daughter, aged six, come home from school and tell me she can't be a princess because she's not Caucasian and blonde – 'Sophie said so' – and my faith wobbles.) If you can't be a princess, or go on *Love Island*, there are plenty of other ways to make a place for yourself in the world, to shape your identity and put a value on yourself. And make that value high. If you don't do it for yourself, no one else is going to. You might be the funny one (though only an idiot would fall for it; funny is our favourite Trojan Horse, often mistakenly conflated with unthreatening), the sporty one, the clever one, the successful one. You might even be all four. How much easier is it to no longer worry about the male gaze being withdrawn if you were never defined by it in the first place? (Although that said, I don't think there's one among us who hasn't, at some point, no matter how unconsciously, fallen back on how we look ...)

The alternative? Stay as appetising and responsive as possible for as long as possible, the subliminal – or not so subliminal – message goes, and you'll be OK. Seriously, who'd be a young woman again, with that to look forward to?

But here's a cheery thought: MILFs are all the rage, according to Candace Bushnell in *Is There Still Sex In The City?* (the answer to which appears to be a resounding no!). 'In 2007 the most googled porn request was MILF,' she says cheerily. 'In other words, there is now a whole generation of young men who've been turned on by the idea, at least, of sex with a woman 20 or possibly 30 years older. And why not? Due to exercise, hair extensions, Botox and filler, healthy eating and advanced skincare, even if a woman is technically too old to bear a child, she can still look like she can.'

But who'd want to? For me, putting an end to waxing, shaving, threading, plucking, tweaking, highlighting, fake-tanning, extending and starving (some of which I never did, and some of which I did a lot), all to look like 'a purse that's been in a fire' (I don't know who I stole this from, but I definitely stole it from someone) is one of the main benefits of menopause. All that 'presenting as female' stuff ... I can't be arsed. It's exhausting. I'm not about to stop wearing makeup altogether (I wouldn't do that to you) but the rest of it, forget it. But that's me. Many of the women I spoke to were reluctant to ease up on the maintenance front – not for fuckability's sake, in the main they weren't very interested in that, but for their own.

'I love that I can make myself look ten years younger with a decent lick of paint,' Paula, 49, told me. 'Basically, Sam, I'm not ready to be old.' Kate, 50, agreed that she wasn't ready to 'stop looking in the mirror.' And Jojo, 50, says she now does more maintenance than ever. 'Now I run a few times a week, I have a personal trainer. I spend a lot of money on skincare, I have my hair done. I do all those things. I just pay a lot more attention.' As does Caroline, 55: 'My waist might be spreading but I'm becoming much better at taking good care of myself.'

Dye or don't dye. Thread or don't thread. Wax or don't wax (although when menopause truly comes, trust me, you're really not going to need to ...), most of the women I spoke to, whether they were 40 or 70, were way past caring whether society thought they were fuckable. What united them, though, was an interest in redefining sexy for a new generation of smart, grown-up women. Women who are done with being told what is and isn't sexy, what is and isn't attractive, what is and isn't sexual and wanted to shape a new identity for themselves.

In *Flash Count Diary*, Darcey Steinke quotes Simone de Beauvoir: 'The ageing woman well knows that if she ceases to be

134

an erotic object it is not only because her flesh no longer has fresh bounties for men, it is also because her past, her experience, make her, willy-nilly, a person; she has struggled, loved, willed, suffered, enjoyed, on her own account. This independence is intimidating.'

I love this. For me, it redefines sexiness and sums up how I'm feeling right now. Not fuckable, as society defines it, but still sexual on my own terms. After decades of having our place in the world assigned to us based on our youth and beauty, decades of contorting ourselves into the boxes society chose for us, being able to decide what and who we want to be feels like being let off a leash. When what you look like is less of an issue, who and what you are is the point. How insanely refreshing is that?

Confidence is sexy. Agency is sexy. Knowing your mind is sexy. Smart is sexy. Funny is sexy. Solvent is sexy. Strong is sexy. Experience is sexy. Being in control of your own destiny is sexy. Breaking a few rules and nobody noticing that you have is sexy. Not caring whether or not you're sexy is sexy.

As for fuckable? Who cares?

'When you talk about menopause, men just die ... a slow death.'

Viola Davis

9

ATROPHY, IT MEANS WITHERING (OR MY LIFE IN LUBES)

If the mere word 'atrophy' makes you want to hide
behind the sofa with your hands over your ears,
you might want to skip this chapter about sexual
dysfunction in perimenopause. Alternatively, gird
your loins, reach for the lube and plough on ...

I'm not going to go into it in glorious technicolour detail: the
dryness and stinging and burning and splitting and itch itch itching. It's too much information – for me and for you (and
definitely for my mum). All I'm going to say about it is that sex
was good, everything was totally 'normal' (whatever that is), if
occasionally a bit on the dry side, and, then, almost without
warning, it wasn't. And then, before very long, it *really wasn't.*
Around about the time I was swimming in sweat all night my
internal lubrication system packed up. Infuriating given how
much liquid the rest of my body seemed able to excrete. Then sex
started to sting and then burn and somewhere in between the
itching kicked in. At first it was easy enough to ignore beyond 20
minutes or so after having sex. A cold bath and no knickers would
see it off. Lubricant made a difference. At first. And then it didn't.

Before long, nothing did. I didn't know this was what 'vaginal atrophy' was until it happened to me. And, let's be honest, if anyone had tried to tell me this could happen, would I have listened? Or would I have turned the page hastily, much as I expect you're doing now?

So let's do away with suspense and cut to the conclusion: I sorted it! Yep, all good now. Ninety per cent good anyway, and that's good enough for me. Thanks to topical oestrogen and hydrocortisone cream and a vat of lube and nothing but cotton underwear for as long as we both shall live. It took years. It started with KY and it ended with KY (#notanadjustafan) and in the middle I encountered (and spent my hard-earned cash on) more lubricants than I even knew existed.

For as long as I can remember we'd used KY, just to help things along, occasionally. It had always done the job when required, but somewhere along the line I realised that it no longer did. Bottom line, I was relying on a tube of chemicals to do what my body no longer would. Or, more accurately, could. And that was *with* HRT.

'KY is too harsh,' the internet experts excoriated me (yes, I know). 'The vulva is too sensitive for that stuff.' 'That shit's got chemicals in,' said someone who was obviously a qualified medic ... Was that true? 'It's possible it's too harsh,' gynaecologist Claire advised. 'Even if it didn't used to be. Tissue changes. You could try something gentler, without glycerin or parabens. Something water-based.' Along with a prescription for oestrogen pessaries, she gave me some leaflets for more 'female friendly' lubricants, and a bunch of sachets to try. We tried the sachets. I can't remember the brands TBH, I only remember that they were less effective than the KY because they didn't actually lubricate. That's the thing, the chemicals and glycerin in the KY may be what make it irritate, but they are also what make it work.

It was much the same with the other lubricants we tried. Now, just because they didn't work for me, it doesn't mean they won't work perfectly well for you. But the thing to remember about water-based lubricants is they're what they say on the pack: water-based. Which means that if they're going to work, they require pretty frequent reapplication. After a while you might as well just be watching Netflix.

I tried several different vaginal moisturisers, too. These are also entirely self-explanatory – they moisturise your vagina. They're not lubricants, they're there to relieve dryness. And, to a greater or lesser extent, that's what they do. I tried a few different brands: big name brands, own brands, random packets picked up in health food shops. Honestly, thinking back, the stuff I stuck in my vagina makes my mind boggle and almost definitely didn't help the long-term irritation prognosis. Self-medication is the curse of women's health and nowhere more so than menopause. I'm a big fan of word of mouth but, really, in this case, screw that, get yourself some expert advice. Even if you have to sell some furniture.

After four or five failed attempts I worked my way along the shelf in Boots and reached Balance Activ Moisture Pessaries Plus. After a couple of weeks inserting those three times a week, usually before bed, there was a definite difference. With that and the KY, things were much better for a while. Until the itching started ... It began at night and for a while I thought it was just part of the night sweats. If you're hot, clammy and sweaty, it's hardly surprising if you're itchy, too. The 3am anxiety attacks were so much worse when there were insects crawling under my skin. At first I was only conscious of it if I woke up because of a night sweat or anxiety attack, but soon it was almost all bloody night. It drove me crazy. During the day, though, it was largely fine. For a while. Then it started to invade my days, too. If I went to the gym, I itched. If I wore tight jeans, I itched. If I went for a long-ish walk, I itched. If I sat too long (by which I mean more than about ten minutes) with my legs crossed, I itched. And then I just started itching randomly throughout the day. Sometimes the itching also burned. What had started in my perineum moved to my labia; the entire area became so sore it started to split. Concentration on anything other than not scratching became impossible. The only thing that worked was a cold bath. And I could hardly sit in a cold bath all day and hold down a full-time job. You know those heat pads you can buy to put inside gloves in winter? Someone should make cool pads to stick in your pants. They'd clean up.

I ditched the pessaries assuming that they were the source of the itch, but the itching didn't go away. I threw away any knickers that weren't cotton. I stopped wearing tight clothes. I stopped using bubble bath and soap. I tried nappy cream, Sudocrem, most of the sensitive-skin shelf in Boots' pharmacy. By this time, you'll be shocked to hear, sex was pretty much out the window. In the end I dragged myself back to Claire, who checked my oestrogen levels (they were fine), asked me about my stress levels (through the roof, as it happened, turns out there was a link – who knew?) and prescribed a hydrocortisone cream to be applied twice daily for two weeks and kept in the fridge. I'm pretty sure it was the fridge bit that was the biggest relief. I would have slept in there if I could.

That was a couple of years ago now. I still use the hydrocortisone cream very occasionally, and KY and occasional applications of oestrogen sorted the rest. Sex is back. I no longer think about my itchy vulva all day every day. Or even once a day. The normality of it is heaven.

Before we go any further, I want to say two things:

1. DO NOT SHOOT THE MESSENGER. I didn't make the rules. This may not happen to you. Some of it might. None of it might. It's a fucking lottery. But to pretend some of it's not crap is BS. Some of it is crap. Some of it is a lot crap. I hope for your sake you don't have to go there.

2. And, as I keep saying but it bears repeating here, that's just me. There were moments when going through perimenopause

felt like being trapped in some kind of computer game – like Indiana Jones and the Vulva of Doom. Yep, it would all be great when I got out the other side. There in the land of zero fucks (giving, not having!) lay freedom, independence, being your own woman. But between me and that lay a pile of shit that felt designed to drive me completely mad. And for a while it did. You will be different. That is the only thing I can 100 per cent guarantee. What worked for me may well not work for you; it's a pricey process of trial and error. Or not. You may not need to go there at all. You may float through perimenopause a little grumpier and come out the other side wondering what all the fuss was about (like my friend Emma). Well, good for you. I'm not remotely bitter.

Anyway, for me, of all the nasty little tricks that sick bastard perimenopause had up its sleeve, this was the very worst: vaginal atrophy. Yep. Vaginal fucking atrophy. (*'Don't say that word!'* more than one of my friends has yelled at me, waving their hands and backing away. Like it's Voldemort or something. But you know what Harry Potter says, fear of the name increases fear of the thing itself.) Or genito-urinary syndrome of menopause (GSM to its friends), as the whole drying, thinning, stinging, burning, night-time vulval itching horror show is apparently now officially known.

Atrophy. What kind of word is atrophy? If you want a one-word ticket to feeling old, you've got it right there.

'A trophy?' another friend quipped on WhatsApp. 'My vagina is a trophy!' Well, yours might be, love, but right now, mine is just grateful to be back up and functioning. But that's the thing, atrophy is such a horrible word that the only logical thing to do with it is take the piss out of it. Otherwise you'd have to confront the fact that it is the very definition of wasting away, for that is its definition. As is 'degeneration of cells', 'becoming vestigial during evolution', 'gradually declining in effectiveness or vigour due to under-use or neglect'. Yes, you read that right. There are English dictionaries that would have you believe that your vaginal dryness etc is the result of your neglecting to use it. Trust me, the atrophy came way before the period of under-use – it was, fairly obviously, the cause of it.

Oh, and while we're lobbing gynaecological grenades around, do you want the good news or the bad news: your pubic hair will eventually thin as you go through perimenopause, but in the case of many women I know the bikini line clings on for grim death while the rest … doesn't. How fucked up is that? For most who take HRT it grows back to a greater or lesser extent, but I can't tell you what colour it will be. (And you thought you'd be glad to see the back of those pubes …) Sorry to be the one to tell you all this, but that's what we're here for, isn't it? The good, the bad and the repulsively ugly of life after 45-ish? Those are all things. Pretty unpleasant things, too. There are moments when it feels like your body and society are conspiring to amplify that feeling of redundancy. And if you're post-menopausal and don't know what I'm on about, don't get too smug because those things are not confined to perimenopause. They can happen when you're post-menopausal too. (Hence the proliferation of acute UTIs in post-menopausal women who don't take HRT or extra oestrogen.) Like I said, don't shoot the messenger. If you want to shoot someone, I can think of a few scientists. Many, but not all, male. Because, you know, they'd obviously know how it feels …

Things to make you cross:

Recent research found that having more sex apparently makes early menopause less likely (there's that 'under-use' thing again). A study of nearly 3000 women, carried out over ten years, found that those who said they 'engaged in sexual activity weekly' (by which I'm assuming they mean intercourse but they don't specify) were 28 per cent less likely to have experienced menopause at any given age than women who did it less than monthly.[18] Megan Arnot, a researcher who conducted the study at University College London, said the findings suggest that if a woman isn't having sex and there is no chance of pregnancy, the body might 'choose' not to invest in ovulation ... (Hang on, sorry, what happened to us having a finite reserve of eggs that varies from woman to woman and runs out when it runs out ...?) So, just in case you didn't feel crap enough already, there's another thing that's your fault.

Well, I'm calling bullshit on that.

It's far from the first time the influence of lifestyle has been argued to be, if not a defining factor in menopause experience, then a significant one. Rama Singh, an evolutionary biologist at McMaster University in Canada, believes menopause doesn't stop women reproducing, it's stopping reproducing that creates menopause.[19] So surely, women like me who have not reproduced at all should be on target for an extremely early menopause indeed, rather than the slightly early 46 I experienced? Unless, of course, we're tricksy and keep having penetrative sex to try to fool it. Because why else would you have sex but to procreate? When you start digging around in this subject it's like being transported back to the 1950s.

Basically it's the health iteration of victim-blaming and has its roots in something called 'psychic insufficiency'[20], which, if you're interested, is a historic notion that if you have a bad menopause it's your own fault. Shades of my nan. All I can say is somewhere along the line I must have been very bad indeed.

If you're not rabid with rage yet, here's one more: In *Emotional Problems of Living*, O. Spurgeon English and Gerald H.J. Pearson argue that women who 'are not enjoying bringing up their children, who are working too hard and taking life in deadly seriousness should have it pointed out to them that if they continue this course they are almost certain to be tired disillusioned people at 50.'[21] I can't even dignify that with a response.

But the bottom line is, science really does seem to be arguing that once you stop using them, your ovaries and associated organs shrivel.

Menopause is an under-researched, under-reported and under-funded project. And nowhere is our ignorance around menopause more enraging than here. There are either as few as 34 or as many as 66 symptoms, depending on which piece of research you believe, and obviously you're not going to get all of them – unless you're very, very unlucky – but one thing everyone is agreed on, hot flushes are the most common. Second most common – the dreaded vaginal atrophy. A study in the International Journal of Women's Health indicated that about 50 per cent of post-menopausal women report at least one symptom.[22]

Someone who experienced all the symptoms was Jane Lewis. Now 54, she's written a book called *Me and My Menopausal Vagina* to share her own experience of extreme vaginal atrophy and her quest, if not to resolve it, then at least to make it possible to live with. It's not exactly public-transport reading – although I feel inclined to give it a go and put the results on YouTube, you'd be guaranteed to get a socially distanced journey – but if you are in a world of pain, there's no other book like it. Her experience of VA (as she calls it) makes mine seem like an occasional itch.

'I'm not quite sure the exact moment when things went so drastically downhill, but I do remember one day being at the cinema and suddenly realising that I couldn't sit down,' she writes. 'After only 20 minutes, I took myself to the back of the theatre and stood alone, swaying from side to side trying to calm the burning. I haven't been able to sit through a film since. If I look back now, I can see that there were already little signs that something was wrong when I was around 45: finding underwear uncomfortable, feeling suddenly very aware of my vulva, getting vaginal ache after a long day standing as a florist. As strange as it now sounds to me, I didn't think anything of it – just getting on with my day, going commando when my vulva felt sensitive and taking some painkillers if I got sore.'

That was only the beginning. 'Who knew it could burn, burn, burn so much?' she goes on. 'Ice packs, heat packs, frozen tins and vegetables all went between my legs in an attempt to calm the flame, and my day revolved around freezing different food items and kitchenware to find the best results.'

Seven years on, Jane has given up her job and has probably seen more medical health professionals than the rest of us put together. 'I've been to counsellors, doctors, nutritionists, physiotherapists, gynaecologists, vulva-dermatologists, pain specialists, urogynae-cologists, sexual health specialists and medical herbalists. I've had acupuncture, hypnotherapy, reiki, spiritual healing, massages, reflexology and CBT. I've tried and applied almost every cream, lubricant and moisturiser there is, spending literally thousands of pounds that I don't have on trying to find "a cure"', she says. 'I wept my way around almost every local park, and had my vagina lasered like a Star Wars lightsaber.'

Ah, the vaginal lasering. Jane was in the last chance saloon when she discovered vaginal lasering. At £1,500 a go and a minimum of three sessions for it to have any chance of working, plus the cost of travel to and from London where the few clinics are, it was expensive but she was prepared to try anything. Even if, in the back of her mind, was the fear it might make her already chronic burning pain worse.

'The idea behind this treatment was that the laser would help to stimulate the production of collagen in the vulvovaginal area, which would therefore rejuvenate the atrophied tissue and spring it back to life,' she explains. 'By plumping it back up, the area would have more elasticity and hydration and would therefore feel less delicate and prone to tearing. Every professional offering the laser treatment claimed it wouldn't hurt and would be only minimally invasive: no surgery, no lasting side effects, and no pain. Other than the price, it sounded too good to be true.'

Jane's story is genuinely excruciating. She makes me feel like a lightweight for moaning at all. (How much of a woman thing is that? Oh, my pain doesn't count because it's not as bad as your pain? Seriously. Snap out of that.) But the upshot is, after a lot of

145

money and several sessions, it was the vaginal lasering that got her back on the path to some semblance of normal life. At least being able to wear knickers every day.

But in what world is this OK? In what world is it remotely acceptable to expect women to 'spend literally thousands of pounds that [we] don't have on trying to find a cure' for something that is so detrimental to our quality of life that it means we don't have one?

Our world. A world where it only affects women. A world where shame and silence are considered effective tools for dealing with 51 per cent of the population.

Jane again, because frankly Jane has been through so much: 'If some of the medical advice I was given in 2018 was to have more sex when my vagina and vulva were so swollen, so red and so sore I could barely walk, there seems to be something very, very wrong with our understanding of the condition and of our treatment of women. I think until we all start talking openly about it ... this expectation of silence and acceptance will only continue, leaving women all over the world feeling ashamed, alone and desperate. Would we give men the same advice if they went to the doctor with a swollen, bleeding and splitting penis? Would we really tell him to have more sex and to just forget about it? Or that it's a normal part of being a middle-aged man? I don't think so.'

There is a serious empathy issue going on here. To say the least. A vast majority of the women I spoke to described their interactions with their GPs in relation to menopause as 'unsatisfactory', 'pointless', 'a waste of time', 'depressing'. Unsurprisingly, those who reported most success talked to female GPs of a similar age. (This is not to take a swipe at GPs – God knows they have more than enough to do, and they can't be experts in everything. Clue's in the name: GENERAL Practitioner. But the default response does seem to be dismissive or judgemental. I talked to women who were refused HRT, as if taking it was some kind of cop out; and women whose GPs wanted to get them off HRT as soon as they got them on it because of the risks (which may well be valid, depending on your perspective, but who made the rule that GPs get the final say?). And there was zero mention of the benefits of topical oestrogen in terms of osteoporosis, UTIs, etc.

George, 51, was told 'we've all got to get older' by a female GP who was 28. Lisa, 52, found her GP's surgery 'useless. They made "poor you" noises, but other than whacking me on HRT there was no other help. It's a major part of a woman's life, yet there's no menopause clinic that encompasses all the aspects of it.' There are menopause clinics, of course – 74 in the UK at the last count – but like everything connected to women's health, it's a postcode lottery: if you know where to look, if you live in the right place, if you can get your GP to refer you, or if you have the ready cash, you can get the treatment. Same old, same old.

There's a pattern here. Many of the women I spoke to who consider their menopause treatment satisfactory or better had sought help privately. Like I did. These are not wealthy women awash with cash, they are ordinary women who'd reached the end of their tether after finding the NHS simply wasn't equipped to help them. As I was writing this, for instance, HRT patches were going in and out of stock like yo-yos. So, too, were the moods, confidence and lives of the poor women who relied on them. Female testosterone is not available on the NHS. Nor is vaginal laser surgery – even for those in extreme need like Jane Lewis. If you want it, you'll have to pay. If you can't pay? Tough. 'It's like they think we're being entitled thinking we should have a quality of life,' laughs George bleakly.

Just because age can, quite literally, wither us, it isn't actually proven to affect desire at all. Many of the women I spoke to said that their libido had crashed since they'd started experiencing perimenopausal symptoms, and they simply weren't interested in sex at all; but in the next breath many said that sex was painful (as a result of dryness) or admitted they were bored to death of their partner. So what comes first, the waning libido or the contributing factors that turn it off? Certainly, my libido was all over the place and there were many weeks, if not months, when my body physically objected and I simply couldn't get my head in the right place. But like the rest of us, and contrary to the bollocks society peddles us, our libido isn't dying, it's recalibrating. Redefining itself. So maybe we just need to reimagine what sex looks like and where and how we direct our desire. Maybe we no longer need or *want* to focus on penetrative sex? After all, what now makes us tick has changed in so many ways, why would our libidos be any different?

As part of her research for her book *Flash Count Diary*, Darcey Steinke attended the 11th European Congress on Menopause and Andropause (age-related hormonal shifts in men) in Amsterdam. There, she reports, a man on a panel 'talks of shrinkage, lack of pliability, dryness. All his descriptions explain how the vagina might feel to an incoming penis. The vagina as a viable penis holder. Not how a vagina might feel to the woman it belongs to.'

This is disappointing, but in no way surprising. You only have to google sex and menopause to see that of the top five most googled things, the fourth is 'a husband's guide to great sex after menopause'. Now, that's important – of course it is, if you're in a loving heterosexual relationship and want to maintain it. Your partner's enjoyment of sex is important in any loving relationship regardless of sexuality. But, erm ... so is yours!

One of the things that really bothered me when I was talking to other women about their sexual relationships with their partners was not how many had totally lost interest – although plenty had – but how many felt they weren't entitled to pull back from penetrative sex with their (male) partner regardless of discomfort, disinterest or downright agony. It wasn't a huge proportion, certainly not as much as 20 per cent. But it was more than ten. 'My partner has a very high sex drive, so we have sex twice a week,' says one. 'Without sex I don't think our relationship would last, as he'd probably look elsewhere.' I wish I could say this remark was a one-off, but it wasn't.

As if it needs saying, the vagina is not a 'penis holder'. What matters first and foremost is how it feels to you, its owner, during sex, sure, but also as you go about your daily business. But that's not the way society works, is it? Society, even now, is penis first.

In *Is There Still Sex In The City?*, Candace Bushnell considers having a type of vaginal laser surgery known as the Mona Lisa treatment after being told by her gynaecologist that 'your vagina isn't flexible enough' – for what she doesn't specify, so I can only presume for a 'penis holder'. (As an aside, this kind of unwanted, unasked for 'advice' is *so* common. When I spoke to her for *The Shift* podcast, French model Caroline de Maigret, 44, told me about a trip to the dermatologist for a regular mole check where she was asked what she planned to do about 'those wrinkles'.) The Mona Lisa treatment, or 'Viagra for girls' as Candace dubs it, somewhat weirdly since it's laser, costs $3,000 a pop and has nothing in common at all with Viagra (£19.99 OTC without prescription at your local chemist) other than it prioritises penetration and the man's experience of sex. Bushnell claims that it's not unusual for a Manhattan husband to give his wife the Mona Lisa treatment for her 50th birthday. It strikes me that's more of a gift for him, than a gift for her.

While I recoil at the thought of having tweakments on my fanny, Jane Lewis's experience did make me pause. For her the surgery (which is not available on the NHS at the time of writing) had a life-changing impact. Her story makes me see there's a time and a place for vaginal laser surgery – but it's not to make sex better for your partner, whatever your sexual persuasion, it's to make life better for you.

Libido is a head thing as much as a body thing. Consequently, the anxiety, confusion, lack of confidence, insomnia, sweats, lack of purpose and poor body image all combined meant that there

149

were days, weeks, even months, when I lost sight of myself to such an extent that I couldn't even spell horny let alone feel it. And though I felt bad about that, my partner was understanding and kind. I've never been very good at talking about sex – I didn't grow up in a house where you just dropped it into conversation, and I always feel like I must be doing it wrong (as with most things in life, so sex isn't special in that regard) – so it took me a while to confront this head-on. Or, to be more honest, it took me a while to let him confront it head-on. Eventually we did and now it's better, more fun, than ever before.

Lisa Diamond, author of the groundbreaking 2008 study *Sexual Fluidity: Understanding Women's Love And Desire*, believes relationship context is particularly important to women, so much so that some 'have suggested reframing "low sexual desire" as a "desire discrepancy" ... after all, maybe a woman's sex drive seems low only when her partner wants sex more often than she does. If that is the case,' Diamond adds, 'who has the problem?!'

We've all had that conversation with our friends where we talk about how for us sex is now more and more in our head and less and less in the groin. 'I feel at our age more than any other, feeling sexy starts in the mind,' says Stephanie, 49, 'and I can't/don't want to just have sex for the sake of it. He doesn't get that obviously and it doesn't matter how much I tell him – and believe me I do.'

But for others it's more serious. For Nahid, 52, it was not so much disinclination so much as repulsion. 'Very simply, I did not want to be touched when I felt I was going mad with the worst symptoms of menopause and so didn't have sex for six to nine months,' she says candidly. 'I just did not want to share my body or be intimate. My husband was very understanding, as we have been together for 20 years and it goes in waves. But I felt I didn't know myself, so certainly didn't want to open up to anyone else physically. Which is my right, I feel, even in a long-standing relationship. I'm getting myself back now and sex is once more enjoyable ...'

Nahid is more in tune with her body than most. Not everyone, even in long-standing loving relationships, feels as comfortable. 'My partner has a high sex drive, so we have sex twice a week,' says Jill, 50. 'I'm not especially needy in this area but I do feel much better when I've had an orgasm. I suffer low self-esteem and body-dysmorphia (made worse by menopause) so I can't understand why he is so keen on me physically! When we do it I do actually enjoy it (a bit like exercise!). Loads of my friends say they're not very active sexually but we're not in the habit of talking about it in detail.'

'Sex has been up and down rather than in and out!,' laughs Stephanie. 'It's been better since I went on HRT, although I might go and talk to the doctor about testosterone.'

Kate, 50, is also considering testosterone. 'I've written about this stuff over the years and I remember doing a piece about five years ago about how all these men – and some women – in the City started taking testosterone in their late thirties and early forties because it gave them the aggressive, willy-waving edge that bankers need, and I remember thinking, "Ooh, I could do with a bit of that." It was when I was in what I now think of as an abusive relationship with various editors and thought I needed to present a stronger impression so they didn't feel like they could fuck with me and not pay me the right fees. So I wanted to take testosterone so I could fuck with people I felt were fucking with me! Which is not very progressive, is it?!'

My friend Clare took it for several months, but stopped when, she says, 'It made me so horny I would have humped a tree. I just couldn't think straight. If that's what it's like being a bloke, no thanks! But I assume I just wasn't given the right dose.' That's possible and made more likely by the fact male testosterone is available on the NHS, but right now female testosterone isn't.

Not everyone experiences a drop in libido when it comes to the menopause. For some it's the opposite extreme. Or both! Writing in *Granta*, Mary Ruefle said, 'You have on some days the desire to fuck a tree, or a dog, whichever is closest.' Caroline, 55, describes hers as sometimes 'raging'. 'There are times when I MUST have sex twice daily and even then it's still biting the inside of my leg,' she says. 'Then suddenly an early night with a lovely book is way more enticing.'

And many of those who do experience a low libido have found talking openly and addressing problems in other areas of their life can kickstart it again. Caroline and her husband of 20 years nearly split up a couple of years ago after she felt she had fallen into the role of unpaid carer and putter-up-with-er. Menopause woke her up to what she describes as her 'subservience and compliance'. She was 'exhausted and furious and menopause gave [her] a surge of strength' that led them to move house and reassess their relationship and their respective roles in it, as well as her husband giving up booze. 'My libido is still quite high, as is his. Mine reached a sort of manic peak around five years ago and has now settled to a nice (probably still quite high) manage-able level. We're fairly active on that score and seem to be pretty matched.'

Many women embark on a wholesale re-evaluation of the role sex plays in their life and their relationship. At 51, and divorced from the father of her children, Betsy Murphy decided to live for a year without any sexual contact with anyone except herself. 'It was inspired by wanting to be able to speak to women authentic-ally about how to keep the body turned on even when you aren't with a partner,' she told me. 'And I didn't want to do it with toys or courses or sessions with "sex experts". In the quest for better orgasms – or any orgasm! – I was someone who took courses and classes and was also seeing many women rushing to sign up for the same "experts" and buy the latest product designed to heal or enhance the vagina (jade eggs! Herbal dildos! Rose quartz dildos! Yoni massages!). I was curious to see what/if I could feel after so many years of feeling nothing.'

After just a month of only having sex with herself, Betsy started to see a difference in how she viewed herself and her body. 'I was finding a shift in my perception of sex and how it was represented in our culture. I wasn't having the sex depicted in movies or porn or romance novels. I wasn't even having the sex I'd experienced with my most favourite partners. It gave me a new meaning of sex and sensuality where it was not just my birthright to feel good in my body – it was also my responsibility to nourish it.'

In possibly the best analogy I have ever heard, Betsy compares her relationship with sex to legendary American cook Julia Child's relationship with cooking. 'I was 32 when I started cooking,' Child said. 'Up until then, I just ate. The measure of achievement is not winning awards. It's doing something that you appreciate, something you believe is worthwhile. I think of my strawberry soufflé. I did that at least 28 times before I finally conquered it.'

'Before I was just having sex,' says Betsy. 'Now I was conquering my erotic energy.'

I'm not suggesting you make like Betsy and have sex with yourself and no one else for a year – although, you could do worse – but there's definitely something in the idea of approaching it like a novice. After all, now sex is no longer about procreation; now pregnancy is no longer the latent fear or spoken wish, the desperate urge, no matter how much birth control you do or don't use; suddenly it ceases to be goal orientated. To return to the Child analogy: it's not about winning (baby-shaped) awards. It's not necessarily about anything, except ... whisper it: fun. Now it's a pastime. Not like any other, of course, such as football, sewing or stamp collecting. It's way more intimate and emotionally loaded than that, but still. As Caroline puts it of her born-again relationship, 'The novelty of being on our own again now the children have all left home has yet to wear off. We are still quite excitable. Sometimes at weekends we nip back to bed in the day.'

Sex in your fifties reminds me of nothing so much as being 15 again but without the fear of unwanted pregnancy or being walked in on by your parents. Finding new and imaginative ways to get off that don't necessarily involve 'going all the way'. Orgasm might be something you have to relearn (if you want to; you might prefer to read a book, or go for a ten-mile walk, and that's fine too). Half the fun is in the trying. Foreplay isn't called fore-play for no reason and maybe menopause is time to put the play back into our sexual relationships. And so what if you have to use a bit more lube?

Part Two:
THE SHIFT

'We all spend our twenties and thirties trying so hard to be perfect, because we're so worried about what people will think of us. Then we get into our forties and fifties, and we finally start to be free, because we decide that we don't give a damn what anyone thinks of us. But you won't be completely free until you reach your sixties and seventies, when you finally realise this liberating truth – nobody was ever thinking about you, anyhow.'

Elizabeth Gilbert, Big Magic

'Before I get started, I just want to know, can everyone see me OK? I have to double check because I'm from Hollywood and women my age tend to be invisible.'

Carrie Fisher

10

INVISIBILITY IS YOUR SUPERPOWER

Yes, I'm the one over here, waving my hand in the air ...

'Excuse me, could I ...'

'Hello, can I have ...'

'Excuse me ...'

By now I have resorted to pushing my silver Amex (not platinum but it's twilight in here, he won't be able to see the difference) in the bartender's carefully averted face. Still nothing. This London bar is not particularly full, but neither is it so rammed that it is legitimate to stand here for ten minutes without being served. And it's not just being served, it's the total absence of anything, not even a flicker of recognition, not an 'I'll be with you in a minute'. Nothing. In all honesty, I may as well not be here. I may as well be invisible. Because, of course, to this twentysomething bloke behind the bar I pretty much am. If he's noticed me at all, he's probably wondering who let their mum out dressed like that.

Not for the first time, I seriously consider whipping off my top and throwing myself across the bar. I'm exaggerating, of course. I wouldn't have done it in my twenties, when I had perky tits and a flat stomach and was in much better shape than I realised. And I wouldn't do it now.

The reality, of course, is that I rarely go to bars where I have to stand up and try to get attention. Like everyone else over 35, I've been choosing venues according to seat availability for the best part of 20 years. But even then I've had to jump up and down and wave both arms in order to get a waiter's attention, while, somehow, the men two tables over (who were probably with women half their age) got waited on just by twitching an eyebrow.

This isn't exclusive to bars. It happens pretty much everywhere, from a social perspective. On the street, people – mainly younger people and mainly men, but women, too – walk into me and through me; they rarely look up and, if they do, they grunt. It's like they don't see me. Once, I even looked down to make sure I was, in fact, there. Kristin Scott Thomas nailed it when, aged 53, she observed: 'I'm not talking about in a private setting or anything. But when you're walking down the street, you get bumped into, people slam doors in your face – they just don't notice you. Somehow, you just vanish.'

She wasn't bitching or moaning or self-justifying, or looking for compliments or reassurance, as some in the media were quick to assume – because God forbid any woman in the public eye might make a comment without an agenda. She was just saying, matter-of-factly, 'Oh look, this is a thing. It happens. Isn't it weird?' And it is. It is a thing. It does happen. And it's really, really bloody weird. The first time it happens, the first time, say, someone walks in front of you in a queue, or serves the person behind you first or lets a door go in your face, and not because they were too busy looking at their phone, it's a shock. I remember standing there, in a shop doorway, as the door swung back at me, expecting a flicker of recognition, some sort of apology, but the bloke ahead just looked straight through me. As if I were a ghost. Like I wasn't there.

Leading up to her 50th birthday, the writer Ayelet Waldman gave an interview to Next Avenue in which she said, 'I have a big personality, and I have a certain level of professional competence, and I'm used to being taken seriously professionally. And suddenly, it's like I just vanished from the room. And I have to yell so much louder to be seen ... I just want to walk down the street and have someone notice that I exist.'

I'm not scaremongering. Nor am I buying into some old-school patriarchal narrative that says women become invisible, to society in general and men in particular, once they hit menopause. It's not about the insidious 'letting yourself go' or looking or behaving any differently. I'm simply stating what I have experienced over the past three or four years. And it's not just me and Kristin Scott Thomas and Ayelet Waldman. Of the 50 or so women I interviewed, more than half said they'd experienced the same thing. Let's call it 'early stage invisibility'.

'I am definitely overlooked in queues sometimes,' says Alice, 51, a journalist. 'I literally said to staff in a fancy coffee shop recently, "Am I invisible?" when they ignored me standing there and asked the young woman behind me for her order. But it's OK. I can go to another fancy café. I did. I have never been back.'

'Try getting served at a bar when you're a woman over 50/55. Good luck with that. You could die of thirst,' laughs Diane Kenwood, 60. 'But in plenty of other ways I either don't feel invisible, or I'm simply so completely comfortable with eyes not automatically swivelling in my direction that I really don't notice or care.'

'I live in a friendly suburb of a friendly city, and the only place I ever experience this is in London,' says Sarah, 69, who says she never felt invisible in her forties and fifties socially *or* at work. ('I worked in education, so there were lots of women of all ages, even when I reached the top jobs.') 'In London it's different; getting served or getting a seat is sometimes difficult. People avoid eye contact, they knock into me on pavements, they queue jump in front of me. I'm not sure that invisibility is an age thing so much as a prevailing cultural phenomenon.'

Sarah could well be onto something. Until the Covid-19

pandemic struck, at least, busy, noisy, self-important and new new new were the currency of the day in the cities that dominate, and for better or worse form, our culture. Certainly in the consumerist West and so-called emerging economies. In her preface to *Life Change*, Dr Barbara Evans wrote: 'Women from countries where age is venerated suffer less physically than other women at the change of life, or menopause. Unfortunately ours is not one of those societies.' She's not kidding. When I interviewed bestselling novelist Elif Shafak last year, she made the point that in Turkey and many other Middle Eastern cultures, older (i.e. menopausal) women are treated better than younger women as they become 'less female'. Activist and FGM campaigner Nimco Ali agreed. 'Menopause is celebrated in Africa,' she said. 'Older women are revered.' But in so-called Western industrialised society, just as men seem to solidify, gaining power, gravitas and silver-fox status (bleugh), lording it over the rest of us with their experience as they hit their fifties, scoring top jobs and huge bonuses, so women seem to fade from sight. Actually, I'll rephrase that. Not so much disappear as *be disappeared*. A survey carried out in 2015 of over 2,000 women over 45 found that more than two-thirds felt ignored when they walked into a room, while 50 per cent said they had been 'shelved' or judged negatively, particularly in the workplace, as a result of their age. This sidelining, or ageing out, or whatever you want to call it, is borne out when you look at the pay gap. Standing at 17.3 per cent for all employees and 8.9 per cent for those in full-time work, it rises to a stonking 28 per cent for women in their fifties.[23] And that's *before* you break it down according to race. Yes, we are paid almost a third less than men, which means we should be downing tools at the end of September every year ...

Some industries are better than others, of course. The media, where I made my home, is not great for representation of any sort (race, gender, age, sexuality and certainly not class). Although it's better now than it was when I started out at the end of the eighties.

(It would be hard not to be.) I was often the only working-class person in the room and, for at least the last 15 years of my career, the oldest woman. (Once I moved to start-up-land I was the oldest person in the room until the investors came on board ...) In a female-dominated industry, I only once had a top-level boss who wasn't a man. Women, as I've written before, had a tendency to disappear in their mid-late forties – if they hadn't already been wiped out by motherhood and childcare, that is ... (If the first baby didn't get them, the second almost always did.) On the plus side, the recent appointment of women to the top jobs at both the *Financial Times* and *The Sunday Times* signals a change for the better. Roula Khalaf is the first female editor in the *FT*'s 131-year history, and Emma Jacobs, 53, is the first female editor on *The Sunday Times* in 108 years. Like I said. Progress. S-l-o-w, but progress. The advertising industry is so notoriously bad that only 12 per cent of creative directors in the UK are women[24]. And who are the ads they're making largely aimed at ...? Yep, you guessed it: 85 per cent of purchasing decisions are made by women ...

Women make up just 24 per cent of partners in US law firms[25] and 26 per cent in accounting firms[26]. I could go on, but it's not like you don't already know all this. Retail is a bit better with notable female figureheads, although like many industries of its ilk, it's invariably staffed by women (young) and run by men (older). When you look at the percentage of those senior women who are a) not white and/or b) over 50, you won't need more than one hand.

Don't believe me? Look around. Where are all the 50-plus women on television, on FTSE 100 boards, in parliament? Yes, we can all name a few: Nicola Sturgeon, Fiona Bruce, Kirsty Wark, Mary Beard, Emma Walmsley at GlaxoSmithKline, Carolyn McCall, Christine Lagarde, John Lewis's chair Sharon White all spring to mind, but you wouldn't lose too many hours of your day making that list. It seems like, despite the lip service paid to diversity of all descriptions, most companies still subscribe to the 'we've got one, we've ticked that box' policy that permeated the business world in the noughties. Wonder how that would work if they applied the same thinking to men called Steve.

But but but. This is making it all sound like a massive downer when that couldn't be further from the truth. Because from where I'm sitting, society taking its eye off us at the point we're at our most powerful, most resilient, most energised (my friend Jude calls it 'purposeful energy' and I couldn't put it better) is often the best thing that could happen to us.

As a journalist and presenter, one of my favourite trivial questions to stick on the end of a question and answer session is this: 'What would your superpower be?' The answers are always fascinating and they give you real insight into what different people consider important – and what they think makes them powerful. I've heard all sorts of answers, from 'hostliness', which is one of my favourites, to being able to fly, teleport and mind-read. All very alpha, apart from hostliness – it won't be any surprise to hear that came from a woman.

For me, my superpower of choice is invisibility, always has been. To a certain extent I put that down to being (nearly) the only ginger in the village. Visibility wasn't a problem, it was *the* problem. As a child I longed not to stand out in class. I never put my hand up, never volunteered, never answered a question if I could help it. I longed to be inconspicuous. I wasn't thinking of the practical benefits – of the tricks I would have played with that superpower, the things I could have got away with when no one was looking, the revenge I could have wreaked! – I just wanted to keep my head down. Now, the reasons are different. Just think of the power invisibility could bring. The ability to operate under the radar, the release from other people's expectations and demands ...

In a world where visibility is the measure by which our achievements are judged: likes, retweets, regrams, followers; the means by which we get a seat at the table (if we're lucky), what are the consequences of not being seen, judged, and questioned (and often found wanting)? Put like that, operating below the radar sounds quite nice, doesn't it? Something to aspire to. As women we spend the bulk of our lives on the sharp end of other people's judgement. Every decision questioned, disapproved of, disdained. So, what would happen if you weren't? What if you didn't feel you had to justify every move and take into account everyone else's opinions? What could you do, who could you be, what could you achieve?

'Part of me feels relieved to not be noticed any more,' says Betsy, 57. 'As someone who was "grabbed by my pussy" many times in my first 45 years of life without permission, it's finally not an issue. When I'm with my 28-year-old daughter, I do notice her getting noticed. Fortunately, she knows to speak up if the attention is negative or disrespectful.'

Alice agrees. 'I definitely lean towards the freedom side of the invisibility debate,' she tells me in an email. 'Freedom to care or not care what people think. Including men and women who may or may not find me likeable or desirable. Freedom to choose my future from relative security: I'm fortunate, I have a house, a husband, health, experience, a good job. Freedom to dress as I choose and avoid harassment unlike my twentysomething daughters.'

Unlike my twentysomething daughters. Every woman I spoke to who was the mother of daughters said the same thing. That, while they were delighted to no longer be subject to the male gaze, they felt more aware than ever of the pressures society placed on the young women in their lives, the 'rent' they seem required to pay just to exist in the 21st century.

That's the thing about being a woman – particularly a young woman, regardless of whether or not you're 'a head turner' (a phrase that came up again and again when I was researching this subject) – your visibility is dialled up to the max; to be visible is to be successful, to be sought after (in life, in work, in love ...) And to do that you have to look a certain way, behave a certain way, play a certain game. While at the same time being blamed at every turn when being obliged to play the game results in unwanted attention. There are times when it can feel that just to exist is to be damned if you do and damned if you don't. Add to that the fact that your life has been ruled by your fertility. Until now. Getting pregnant, trying not to get pregnant, being pregnant, not being pregnant, giving birth, being on maternity leave, coming back from maternity leave, bringing up children, juggling childcare, being asked if you're having any more children, being asked when you're going to have children, being asked why you haven't had children, being asked if you *can't* have children, being asked if you regret not having children ... And, not exactly overnight, but in a reasonably short space of time, all of that is gone. Not only the unspoken social rule that says you are somehow entitled to ask any woman, no matter whether or not you really know her, the most intimate details of her reproductive life. (And in the case of pregnant women, touch them.) But the necessity to smile sweetly and put up with it; to answer; to prove anything to anyone. To stick to the prescribed narrative that goes husband, baby, nice house, repeat. Or to justify why you're not sticking to it.

With menopause comes an end to all that. So, you could see this moment as society handing you your P45, or you could see it as being freed up to do other, more interesting things. A time to throw a bloody big party, frankly. Don't look at what menopause takes away, look at what it brings. Because with it, age brings a gift, the same gift Harry Potter received on his first Christmas at Hogwarts. The gift that enabled him to cause even more trouble than the Marauder's Map: a cloak of invisibility. And, now, you have one, too; an aura that allows you to pass unseen under the noses of 50 per cent of the population. (In fact, make that more than 50 per cent because those blinkers aren't gender specific and there will be plenty of younger women who behave as if they can't see you, too.)

'It's a goddamn relief,' Sue, 49, told me. 'For some reason (stemming from my childhood, I'm sure), I've always felt I needed to work really hard to be heard and noticed, and as a woman approaching 50 in the next month, I feel freeeeeeeee. I genuinely couldn't give less of a shit. Invisibility is a welcome relief.'

Of course, a lot depends on who we're invisible to. 'Ducking that world-weary male gaze is a gift,' says Joy, 47. 'I used to turn strangers' heads but now I have a new space to think about how I want to present myself and who I want to be and whether I want to engage at all. I'm gifted choice. Most importantly, I'm still seen by people who love me.'

Sailing under the radar of the male gaze seems to be a problem for precisely no one. 'Frankly, I don't give a shit that I don't turn the heads of men any more,' says Paula, 49. 'But I do care that a woman will sneak up and ask where my shoes are from! If that didn't happen any more, that would be the worst invisibility to me.'

'Am I invisible when I walk into a room? Yes, probably, but it's fine,' says Caroline, 55. 'I never felt particularly "visible" in that scenario when I was younger. I feel happier and more confident in myself these days and more comfortable going up and chatting to people at parties and work dos. That used to strike fear into me. And TBH I'm relieved that the tiny amount of catcalling I endured as a younger woman has now fully died away. I still shudder at the memory of the man on the scaffolding who, in 1983, yelled at me, "Your arse is like two footballs!" I was 18 and wanted to die. I went home and threw away my skinny jeans that night.'

Choice is a gift, if only we let ourselves take it. 'I can be invisible but by choice,' says Alice. 'At work it's a superpower, my male colleagues don't expect me to be quite so feisty. My former boss (a fortysomething woman) told me she was amazed how fearless I was in big work meetings. I think that's partly me always being quite bold but definitely partly just having no fucks to give any more about their opinion.'

That said, Alice, who works for a large corporation, says she feels increasingly invisible when it comes to promotion opportunities. 'I was told last month that a younger colleague had "done more extras", which was simply not true but it made me realise that my "extras" are invisible. I just do them. I don't go on about it. And it's been that way for about five years. Six maybe?' In other words, since she turned 45.

Invisibility isn't an issue for Paula, but she does admit that, as she works in a sales environment, she's conscious she has 'a limited number of years left. The industry I work in likes knowledge and experience but when it reaches the point where my kids could be my clients, it might become harder for me.' She doesn't say whether the same applies for men, but the law of averages suggests not. I also keep hearing 'old enough to be their mum' (words that echoed in my own head constantly when I worked on The Pool). But I've never once heard the same said of men. 'Old enough to be their dad'? Think about it.

'I don't feel invisible ...' Paula continues. And then pauses. 'Yet ... I know it's coming. I still feel confident at work and well respected. I'm very vocal and position myself and play the bollocks politics but I've noticed I have fewer recruiters contact me about other opportunities. In fact, in the last year I've had one, where normally I'd have four or five at least. I'm considered too expensive or too experienced (read: too old).'

That struck a personal chord. Not that long ago I was told that I 'didn't fit the brief' for a big media job. I was then told by someone else, who obviously did, that the brief was '"probably male" with enough gravitas to impress the proprietor'. The person who got the job had almost exactly the same CV as me. The only difference was balls. By the same token, I know of three women aged between 48 and 56 who were 'aged out' of their substantial jobs (how much do I hate the phrase 'aged out'?) in the last six months. Between them they had 90 years of experience. Fortunately they also had good lawyers and rock-solid contracts. Another friend who has run global fashion chains now finds herself 'too experienced' to get 'one of the big jobs'. As Paula said, 'too experienced' is often shorthand for 'too expensive'. Especially if you're female. Who among us hasn't been told: 'We'd love to have the benefit of your wisdom but we don't have the budget to pay you. Can you do it pro bono?'

Bollocks politics indeed.

Women over 50 form one of the largest groups in the Western world. Make that women over 40 and it's THE largest. By the time the oldest millennial turns 50 in 2032, the 50+ market will drive more than half of the US GDP. Think how different things could be if we liked ourselves, harnessed our power, stood up for ourselves, spoke out. 'There is no point in growing old unless you can be a witch, and accumulate spiritual power in place of the political and economic power that has been denied you as a woman,' argues Germaine Greer in her menopause tome *The Change* (written in 1991 but updated in 2018). 'We are supposed to mind our own business. If we are to do this, we need to find business of our own.'

Well, now many of us are and it's changing the world. Let's go back to the list of 50+ women in traditional positions of power we started with earlier. But let's change the parameters a bit. As well as women running countries and FTSE 100 companies – of whom, it's a surprise to no one, there are woefully few – let's add women who are doing their own thing in their forties, fifties and beyond; rather than operating within the restrictions posed by the establishment, let's look at women starting their own. *Then* the list really starts to grow.

Off the top of my head: Natalie Massenet, whose Net-a-Porter threw the world of luxury retail into turmoil because (who knew?) a woman in her forties had a few ideas about how other women might like to shop; Sharon Horgan, who is responsible for some of the most button-pushing comedy writing of the past decade with *Pulling*, *Catastrophe* and *Divorce*, and is transforming TV with the production company she co-founded, Merman; Reese Witherspoon who started her own production company, Hello Sunshine, because she didn't like the roles women were being offered in Hollywood blockbusters and wanted to tell women's stories; Michelle Obama who is basically using being Michelle Obama brilliantly to make the world a better place; Jane Shepherdson, who after decades working for the worst man in retail, Philip Green (and God knows he had some competition), went on to shock the high street by giving women's clothes pockets at Whistles and is now at the vanguard of the fashion rental revolution; Mary Portas, who has reconfigured her business in the image of her 'Work Like A Woman' ethos; Former ad agency executive Cindy Gallop, who has made it her business to call out all the inequalities that permeate her industry; Caryn Franklin, Shonda Rhimes, Val Garland, Jo Malone, Bernardine Evaristo, Jo Whiley, Tracee Ellis Ross, Kate Mosse, Sandra Oh, Gwyneth Paltrow, Dame Stephanie Shirley, Elizabeth Gilbert ... This is by no means exhaustive. In stark contrast to the previous list, I could go on and on and on.

Why? For the same reason minority women now head up almost half of female-run start-ups in the US[27]: ignored and undervalued by the dominant infrastructure, they're used to having to find workarounds. Rather than asking for a seat at the table, they are building their own table. While these women might not be visible to the people who wrote the rules – who are largely white and male – they are to the rest of us. They are doing things their way, operating below the radar and outside the system. They didn't like the rules so they made their own, quietly, tenaciously, and they did it all while no one else was paying attention.

Being at best underestimated, at worst totally ignored may sound familiar. It also sounds like a massive opportunity.

'I felt more invisible from the age of 22 to 39 when I worked in large organisations than I ever have in my forties and fifties. Unless my mainly male colleagues were looking at my tits or my arse, I may as well have not been in the meeting (or even the building) during the years I climbed the corporate career ladder,' says Joanna Davies, who walked away from corporate life and set up Black White Denim almost ten years ago. 'Setting up my own business at the age of 43 made me wholly visible. I'm in a customer-facing business and have had to make myself known to colleagues in the trade, press and, of course, my social media audience. Being invisible is not an option. I took the opportunity to redefine myself, my career and my life and it's ACE!'

As Joy said earlier, the question is 'who exactly are we invisible to?' And, equally importantly, do we care?

Diane Kenwood left a job she loved in her late fifties and has since set about completely reinventing her career. 'It has been invigorating, exhausting, confusing, challenging and enjoyable in roughly equal measure,' she says. 'Being far more invisible in terms of my profile in the world has been a major adjustment and for a long time when anyone asked me what I do, I told them what I used to do. My work calling card had considerable currency and that's where I feel the impact of any invisibility.'

I have to put my hand up here and say I physically winced when I read that line in her email. As editor-in-chief of *Cosmopolitan* and then *Red* I was used to people answering my emails, seeking me out, giving a toss what I thought. I was so used to it that, to my shame, I took it for granted. That'll learn me. When I left, aged 46, and perimenopause came rushing in, it was like tumbleweed in my inbox. The same thing happened after The Pool folded. After decades of being professionally sought after – if only because you are gatekeeper to a platform that others are keen to access – it takes a world of self-confidence, that for a long time I didn't have (and on some days, still don't), to separate who you are from what you did and reclaim some space in the world just for you. There were days (weeks) when it was all I could do to get out of bed. (I remember meeting Elizabeth Gilbert at a drinks party to introduce her novel *City of Girls* and blithely telling her that this was the first time I'd left the house in two months and I was wearing the same clothes I'd been wearing since Christmas. It was March. Obviously I was still quite out of it. Being Elizabeth Gilbert, she smiled at me kindly and said that sometimes just getting out of bed was enough.) It took time to start to believe that regardless of whether society thought it had finished with me, I haven't finished with it.

'I have used my fifties to take control of my life and have a renewed confidence in doing my own thing,' says Genevieve, 57. 'I have also found that the knowledge I've acquired through the years is valuable in a work situation and have been able to use my expertise to an advantage. Specifically, it has opened new doors. When I left my job at 53 I was able to do a bit of writing and presenting as a 50+ expert in beauty and wellness, an area I love ... But I also love imparting advice to others who may find this age challenging in certain respects.' Genevieve has also started 'a 'live TV' career at the grand old age of 57. 'We are lucky in the beauty/wellness industry that it isn't *quite* so ageist. There are many really great, highly respected senior people of 45+ – and also I'm not prepared to take it lying down!'

It's a sentiment borne out by Rowena, who is also in the throes of setting up her own business. 'I definitely don't feel invisible. If anything, I've become more confident, more "me". I care less about conforming or fitting in. I've been self-employed for a while now and I don't feel discriminated against because of my age. If anything I have a lot more to offer now than I did ten, even five years ago. I have more experience, more wisdom and gravitas than I did in my thirties and forties.'

'What if,' to quote Greer again, 'turning 50 gave us the keys to the city ... entitled us to first place in the queue?' I think we can go further than that. What if we build not just our own table, but our own companies, our own city, cut our own keys ...? What's the point of persistently battering on a door that opens to you only reluctantly, and on the rare occasions it does, it contains doors within doors that are only visible to those with balls?

Ageing isn't the worst thing that can happen to a woman. By now we have all lost enough friends, family, colleagues and acquaintances to know what that is. So how about we stop behaving like it is? And instead we grasp the things it brings us: wisdom, experience, an astonishing ability to move mountains while nobody's looking, because the male gaze, like the eye of Mordor, has moved on. And so can we. The invisibility bestowed on us by the old-school narrative that's intended to dismiss us is actually to our advantage. We have the experience that comes from having lived life with all the good, the bad and the ugliness that brings; we've been pulled apart and put ourselves back together again; life might not have worked out how we thought, but we're still standing. Many far better than standing. We have fewer demands on our time and money, and, believe it or not, we have power (oh, yes, we do!), the power that comes from experience and knowing ourselves better than ever. So what if you're 'bossy' or 'difficult' or all those other things women have always been accused of? It's called knowing your mind and standing up for yourself. Get used to it. And, in the immortal words of almost every woman ever, 'I love it when they underestimate me.' Because I promise you that if you don't think you've been underestimated before, you will be now. And while they're not paying attention, you can do whatever the fuck you like right under their noses in a way that you never could while there was (all kinds of) rent to pay, coffee to make and managing up to do.

And really, I don't know about you, but I've just reached a point where I no longer give that much of a fuck what anyone thinks. (Of course, I *do*. But on a good day, with the wind behind me, I only give a fuck about the people and things who really matter to me.) After a life spent in boxes – school boxes, work boxes, ill-advised relationship boxes – trying not to touch the sides, scared of what might happen if I do, you know what I've realised will happen? Nothing. Those walls? Give them a kick. They're made of cardboard, paper-thin. That's why the pale, male and stale don't want to see us. They know that if we do our own thing for long enough, their boxes will start to wobble and collapse. Visibility is in the eye of the beholder, and looking around me I see so many women who are so much bigger than those boxes. Stronger, smarter, more resilient – we just have to allow ourselves to be. Don't worry about invisibility, that's our superpower. All that's stopping us is fretting about it. And when we do, we can get on with the second half of our lives.

I'm giving the last word to Jane Fonda (well, Jane Fonda's character in *Grace and Frankie*) because in my view, the last word should almost always be given to Jane Fonda. 'We have a super-power,' she says, after the two women have been ignored in favour of a young blonde while trying to buy a packet of cigarettes. 'If you can't see me, you can't stop me!'

What are we waiting for?

'When a woman finally learns pleasing the world is impossible, she becomes free to learn how to please herself.'

Glennon Doyle, Untamed

11

ME ME ME

How to say no after a lifetime of saying
yes. A people-pleaser pushes back

'Can you come to this meeting?' *No.* 'Yes.'
   'Are you free on Saturday night?' *No, I'm watching* Spiral. 'Yes.'
   'Can I borrow your black jacket?' *No.* 'Yes.'
   'Would you like pizza?' *No.* 'Yes.'
   'Have you got five minutes?' *No. I don't have five seconds.* 'Yes.'
   'Can you pick me up?' *No.* 'Yes.'
   'Make me a coffee while you're at it.' *Sod off.* 'Sure.'
   'Can I have next week off?' *No.* 'Yes.'
   'You can cover that presentation for me, can't you?' *No.* 'Yes.'
   'Can I borrow a hundred quid. I'll pay you back.' *I've heard that*
before. 'Of course.'
   'Do you want to come to this launch with me?' *No.* 'Yes.'
   'Chinese or Indian?' *Indian!* 'Up to you.'
   'Can I pick your brains?' *No.* 'Of course.'
   'Do you mind if we rearrange?' *Yes.* 'No problem.'
   'Can you host this event for a quarter of your usual fee?' *No.*
'Oh, go on then, as it's you.'
   Every single time I want to say no, I start to worry about
inconveniencing the person doing the asking. Or upsetting them.
Or, worse, disappointing them. (How much do I hate that word,

the bane of my life: I'm not cross, I'm just – pause for effect – *disappointed*.) Or letting the side down. Or never getting offered another job. Or I assume I'm in the wrong. Or I feel guilty. Or inconsiderate. Or they won't like me and I want them to like me. (I *need* them to like me.) Or I'm being unreasonable. Or or or. But worse, I *imagine* I know what they want me to do – or at least I try to guess, who knows if I'm guessing right – and then I do it. So, what I'm doing or saying I could actually be doing or saying wrong anyway. Exhausted yet? I am.

Sometimes, it's no big deal. What's another coffee? Even if you paid for the last four (because you are not no way definitely not counting). But on other occasions, my head and heart are screaming, 'Hell no!' but still my mouth opens and I hear 'yes' coming out. I thought I'd found a solution when journalist and author Sathnam Sanghera wrote on Twitter that when he's asked to do something, he always asks himself, 'Would I want to do this if it was right now?' If the answer is yes, he says, he agrees. If not, he doesn't. Simple. Great idea, I thought. Genius! I tried it the next time I was asked to attend an event. I imagined myself doing it. Ugh, I thought. I'd rather watch Netflix and have a takeaway. (Which TBH is true of almost anything I'm asked to do.) I imme- diately started thinking up convoluted ways to get out of it. (I do that a lot.) And you know what I said? Yes. I know. FML. But this is my life. Or it was, until about 18 months ago. And I feel pretty sure it's your life, too. Saying yes. Bending over backwards. Working out what other people want us to do and trying to do it. It's what little girls are trained to do, after all.

I've been trying to pinpoint the first time I did it; the head says no, mouth says yes, thing. Was it at a family gathering, as a small girl of six or seven, maybe eight, already becoming aware that, though her wishes often remained unspoken, my nan's passive aggressive demeanour made it perfectly clear what she wanted you to do? And, more than that, she expected you to do it. (And, God knows, I have never met anyone before or since who could sulk like she could if you didn't.) Was it at primary school, where I realised that people liked you more – or at least tolerated you – if you agreed with them and went along with what they wanted to do? Was it just generally, at home, when I found life was easier all round if I didn't get into trouble? When I cast my mind back I can see hundreds, if not thousands, of incidents; images flickering cine-camera style of little Sam nodding and smiling and doing and helping, one eye on the person asking to make sure that I was getting their approval. My ambivalent relationship with authority figures goes back to an early age. The truth is, the impulse to please wasn't conscious. It was learnt. It was what the world expected. And then it became instinctive. Driven more by the fear of the repercussions of disagreeing or not doing as I was told or, worse, doing it badly – of, and this is crucial, not being a 'good girl' – than by asking myself what I wanted to do, or what I thought, or whether I agreed and acting accordingly.

I pestered my mum for a bra long before I needed one because everyone else had one. I started fancying boys at school because everybody else did. And – although it pains me to say it – that probably goes for losing my virginity, too. At 15, when I was swimming competitively and training every day, I realised that while the exercise had seen off the puppy fat that had plagued me since I was a child, it had also turned my already-wiry red hair to straw. I turned my attention to my appearance and didn't like what I saw. Exams were on the horizon. Everyone else had boyfriends. My skin and hair looked like I spent an hour submerged in chlorine every day (because I did), so I decided something had to give. The swimming went. It went because that was what I thought I wanted at the time. But now, I look back and see it was what I thought I *should* want. Like the first boyfriend who was the captain of the school football team and the thigh gap you could measure in inches and the eyelashes half an inch long, instead of the stubby fair ones I'd been born with, and the poker-straight blonde hair that eludes me to this day.

Because in the hierarchy of our school, those things would give me far more acceptance than straight As ever had.

For me, that time, 13 to15, was pivotal in persuading me to climb into my box, a box that would get – for a while – ever smaller. This is not specific to me. This is the case – to a lesser or greater degree – for pretty much every woman I know. (I'm inclined to say every woman below 50, certainly below 60, but I'm leaping ahead, so hold that thought for a page or two.)

American activist, speaker and bestselling author Glennon Doyle puts that pivotal age a little younger. She pinpoints ten as the age when she submerged her sparky little girl self and learnt to be a good girl instead. 'Ten is when we learn how to be good girls and boys,' she writes in her memoir-cum-call-to-arms *Untamed*. 'Ten is when children begin to let go of who they are in order to become what the world expects them to be. Ten is when our formal taming begins. Ten is when the world sat me down, told me to be quiet, and pointed to my cages ... I wanted to be a good girl, so I surrendered to my cages. I chose a personality, a body, a faith and a sexuality so tiny I had to hold my breath to fit myself inside.'

She says 'girls and boys' and that's undoubtedly the case for many born to the label 'boys' who don't find themselves fitting comfortably into the straitjacket society puts on them. But in the main we're talking about girls here. Doyle goes on to relate a telling anecdote about her 17-year-old son. He and his friends – a mixed group of teenagers – were hanging out in her TV room. When she asked if anyone was hungry, the boys all said yes without even tearing their eyes from the screen. The girls ... they cast around, eyed each other, telepathed among themselves and then one girl smiled politely and spoke for them as one: 'We're fine, thank you.'

'The boys checked inside themselves. The girls checked outside themselves,' Doyle says. 'We forgot how to know [ourselves] when we learnt how to please.'

That line brought me up short. I recognised it. I recognised it so hard it hurt. Who hasn't done that? Instead of going with your instinct and answering how you see fit – whether it's if you want a burger or don't want a lift home or to swap the late shift at work or to go to that bar where you know you won't get a seat or get served – you cast around, try to work out what other people are thinking and fit in with them accordingly. I can see myself doing it. Again and again and again.

This was me. For most of my adult life. (In therapy it's called hypervigilance and I still catch myself doing it. Watching for an expression. A tightening of the lips. A slip of the eyes. And I instantly wonder what I could have said or done differently to get a different reaction.) It's exhausting and a waste of life. And I have borne the consequences. As have others around me. But not any more. And you know when it stopped? It stopped about three years ago. It stopped along with my periods and HRT – oh, and 18 months or so of therapy. So I'm not attributing the end of my people-pleasing ways wholly to menopause, and the gradual withdrawal of oestrogen, because of course the therapy more than played its part. But I do credit the menopause with finally – 30 years too late – prompting me to seek the therapy I'd needed for so long.

Whether you put it down to the hormone shift and reduction in oestrogen (the biddability hormone, the nurturing hormone or what Dr Julie Holland in *Moody Bitches* describes brilliantly as 'the whatever you want honey' hormone); or that perimenopause 'rewires' women's brains, as Louann Brizendine, author of *The Female Brain*, argues, to make us less nurturing, less willing to put ourselves second and more likely to say 'Sod that!' Or the so-called empty nest syndrome, where after 30 years of focusing on other people – Kids! Colleagues! Partner! Boss! – suddenly you can focus on you. It's not just that the child-wrangling days are behind for those who had children to wrangle (because, let's face it, for many the parent-wrangling days are about to begin), it's that the nurturing imperative that oestrogen is meant to bring is gone.

The upshot is the same: you stop bending over backwards to please others and gradually find you're starting to please yourself.

This is something that arises in almost every book and article I've ever read about the menopause. In *The Change*, Germaine Greer describes it as a sort of return to adolescence. 'The passionate idealistic energetic young individual who existed before menstruation can come on earth again if we let her.' In *The Middlepause*, Marina Benjamin finds herself starting to care less and less. 'In middle age I am discovering that I care less about what other people think. I care less about material things, too – about acquisition more generally.' In 'There Won't Be Blood' in the *New Statesman*, Suzanne Moore celebrates the end of the obligation of 'social lubrication'. 'Use lube for sure. But know that you no longer have to be it. All those years when femininity was enacted as social lubrication have gone. You don't have enough time left to go around making everyone else feel comfortable.' While in *The Bitch Is Back*, a book of essays about mid-life edited by Cathi Hanauer, writer Pam Houston finds herself occasionally withdrawing from friends and acquaintances. 'Mild misanthropy may simply be a thing intelligent women of a certain age grow into because most have spent a huge percentage of their lives taking care of other people.'

But my favourite description of all is by comedian Cally Beaton, writing in the *Guardian*: 'After a five-decade gestation, I've given birth to a darling little bundle of self-esteem.'

Yes! Yes! Yes! After decades of not having the self-confidence, the self-belief, the self-esteem, the self-anything to say, 'No, I don't want to do that,' the end of fertility has brought with it an inner core, if not of steel then of something stronger than whatever was there before. It's given me a backbone of sorts. Life is frankly too short not to have the gumption to express a preference for curry over noodles.

Genevieve, 57, has seen a definite change in her personality over the last few years. 'I think menopause added to this in terms of not suffering fools, not taking shit. That's one of the reasons I left my full-time job.' Me too! 'Additionally, the wisdom that comes with age also allows us to start questioning our friendships. Does that person make me happy? Do I look forward to seeing them – if not, why am I doing it? We all have people in our lives who perhaps shouldn't command the power over us that they do, and this is something I'm trying to take control of. It's not easy but now when I think, "Oh, I haven't spoken to that person in a while, I should call them," I say to myself, "NO I don't need to call them. And NO I don't need to see them."'

After decades of being expected – by society, by our friends and families, by our bosses, by ourselves – to behave a certain way, giving ourselves permission to step back might sound easier said than done. But it's possible and most of the women I've spoken to regard it as absolutely essential. They always did. Only now they're prepared to lay claim to it.

'I've definitely got less people-pleasey in my mid-forties,' says June, 46. 'I recognise the people-pleaser in me a lot more and I call it out in myself when I see it. I think I've got my personal life in pretty good shape. I've stepped away from the life Hoovers and toxic relationships. This has made a huge difference. The only times I find myself falling into it are at work.'

Work is an area where most of us are less confident about speaking our minds. 'I am always saying yes to more than I should,' says Julie, 56. 'I have currently been pushed into looking after the CEO as his PA has left. I don't have the time, nor the inclination. I have enough to do without doing that as well. It's been a recurring theme throughout my life, possibly because I was the eldest child and my dad, particularly, was quite keen on us doing well, so I felt a bit of pressure there. As I've got older, I have got better at saying no, but still say yes far too often – especially on the work front.'

For Shelley Silas, her 60th birthday was a big milestone. 'As I approached 60 I found that I had nothing to prove to anyone,' she says. 'I put myself first mostly, my wife and mum are priorities, too, and I am there for friends who need help, but I have been saying "No" to many things for a while now. I found that I was taking on too much for others, saying, "Yes, I can do that," for the simple reason that I *could* ... and then berated myself because I had no time for my own work and myself and blamed others when it was entirely my own fault! It's been a lesson in the making ... but now I have no problem saying no.'

I thought I was doing well, but some of the women I spoke to for this chapter are absolute legends.

Caroline, 55, has become hardcore both in her work and her private life. 'I was such a pleaser when I was younger, managing an office of 25 people and wanting to be everyone's friend. Probably *the* best aspect of reaching this age is no longer caring so much; not putting everyone else first to the detriment of myself.

'I made the decision last year to renegotiate my contract and basically cut my work right down. It had become the norm for me to take work on every holiday and work late nights/weekends and I was burned out. I won't work like a maniac any more – unless I want to. I won't do shite, badly paid work. I won't do work I'm ashamed of. I'd rather do without.

'Before I agree to a job I have three criteria and it must fulfil at least one. I ask myself:
- Is it easy?
- Is it really well paid?
- Is it fun?
If it's none of those I won't do it.'

Caroline is just as brutal in her private life. TBH I think she should start running masterclasses.

'I won't spend my valuable spare time going to things I don't want to. If an acquaintance wants to stay for the weekend

– basically foisting herself on us, boring the tits off us with her relentless anecdotes – she gets a "Sorry, we can't do that." No big explanation necessary. As for the friend whose attitude towards women was frankly becoming *very* creepy – I explained that I didn't want to see him any more. It felt weird – I had never cut ties with a friend in adult life. But he was draining me and when I realised I had to get drunk in order to get through his visits – well, they had to stop. His feelings are hurt but I couldn't bear his lechy creepy attitude.

'I don't do very much in life that I don't want to do,' she admits. 'The exception is my kids – I'd pretty much do anything for them!'

The great thing about Caroline and Karen, 50, (below) is that they have found practical coping mechanisms for turning their people-pleasing on its head. I'm sharing them because I found them so useful that I figured you would, too.

'People-pleasing was my default setting for so many years,' says Karen, who became estranged from her mother after her father died in 2017, a process she describes as 'really difficult, but [it] began a path to wider life-boundary setting. She describes her life now as 'calmer, more fulfilled, with incredible people in it ... and simpler.'

That said, 'My first reaction to most requests remains fear of saying no,' Karen admits. 'Of disappointing, of being judged, but since going freelance ten years ago, I have incrementally ignored my first reaction and slowly built a work and personal life based on what works for me. At work I have set days in London and I'm only available those days, I try to turn meetings into calls wherever possible, and I always ask for a fair fee. I'm prepared to walk away when it isn't. I've also started resigning clients where their behaviour is unreasonable. For years I felt I should be grateful for the job. Not any more. At home, I have edited my group of friends to a group of us who are honest and equal in our support of each other. None of us gives or asks too much.'

Accommodating others, putting them first, is so ingrained that even those who say they've got much better at it still admit to ambivalence. 'I read Sarah Knight's book *The Life-Changing Magic of Not Giving a F**k*,' says Jenny, 48, 'and while there were elements of it that I completely agreed with, for me it jarred. I found it just *too* self-centred and I wholeheartedly believe there are times when you do have to make sacrifices. You do have to accommodate people you wouldn't necessarily choose to. That's how we build societies and communities and families.'

Then she goes on to tell me about a friend she can't bring herself to cut ties with. 'She's so negative about everything. If we go out for a meal and it's been beautiful and we've had a laugh and then they took for ever to bring the pud – that is what she'll talk about on the way home. The pud being fucking late.' 'Sometimes I think, so this is it, is it? You're going to keep accepting invitations and going out with her and hating it, just because she was kind to you for a very specific part of your life? And at the moment, the answer seems to be yes. I can't make bloody sense of it, I really can't.'

I can. We've been doing it for decades. It's not going to change overnight. But deciding what really matters to you and putting those things front and centre of your life, is not selfish it's not self-centred: it's what millennials call self-care. Try it. It's not something women are trained to do, but when we do, it's a liberation.

For me, the ultimate in self-care is not going out when I don't want to. (Which is not to say I didn't want to with every core of my soul after being in lockdown for months earlier this year.) A committed introvert – or maybe just anti-social – I've spent a lifetime forcing myself to go out when I really wanted to stay in with a boxset (or the testcard, depending on the decade ...). Not bothering to socialise when you can't be bothered to socialise has been my ultimate gift to self. I hate birthday parties and, apart from my 18th, have never celebrated a 'big birthday', although some of my favourite people are fans of fancy dress, so it takes all sorts. On my 53rd birthday I was in

Edinburgh house-hunting, so to 'celebrate' I posted a David Lynch quote on Instagram that said, 'I do go out. I just don't like it.' Nothing could have summed up my attitude to socialising more. The reaction was instant. Hardly anyone likes going out, apparently. They just pretend to because they feel they have to. It was the same when I wrote a blog about how much I love being cancelled on at the last minute – especially in the evenings so I could stay in with a bottle of wine and a boxset. Everyone agreed. Given the choice, people love staying in. It doesn't mean you stop doing all the things that push you out of your comfort zone – far from it; the very fact of menopause is one big *dis*comfort zone – but one of my favourite things about getting older is the fact I can stop pretending to enjoy compulsory socialising. By which I mean going to large social gatherings where I know hardly anyone, not hanging out with friends. Sometimes I go, sometimes I don't. Sometimes I drive by. Sometimes I even stay for a while. And then, when I've had enough, I get my coat and leave. (In fact, I often hang on to my coat to make an Irish goodbye easier. Thanks Marian Keyes for that little gem.) That's the beauty of The Shift.

'We tend to reduce self-care to scented candles and bubble baths,' says Joy, 47. 'Something to buy, something to do. It's really more fundamental than that. It's living well in the space we've got, in the time it takes, day after day. It's something to reclaim, not something to do.' Or, as a shaman who Kate Spicer interviewed for a feature she was writing said, 'Inseminate yourself!'

'I guess you can become your own lover,' Kate laughed by way of translation. 'I don't mean in terms of masturbation – although you can do that – I just mean treat yourself nicely, take yourself out, treat yourself like the princess you wish other people would treat you like.'

As Audre Lorde famously put it, 'Caring for myself is not self-indulgence, it's self-preservation.'

If you're still not convinced, think back. Did Caroline sound selfish or indulgent or did she sound admirably switched on?

Fashion editor, activist and campaigner Caryn Franklin, 61, describes this as a process of re-evaluation, quality not quantity. Quite simply: listening to herself, her body, her hormones and acting accordingly. 'As a result I'm no longer buckling under the stress of numerous projects running concurrently ... I attend fewer time-wasting meetings, engage in much less unwaged work and collaborate more selectively. I'm thinking about the bigger picture as I celebrate my strengths and focus on the positives, while gracefully accepting my limitations ... finally,' she writes on Refinery 29. 'Now, for the first time, free of hands-on child-wrangling, I'm in an intense relationship with myself. It's a joy, as the voice inside me grows stronger and more enquiring of new perspectives ... Shedding old ways and reframing people's perceptions of me, I left the people-pleaser behind. This has been an act of common sense.'

Big or small, self-care has been a lifesaver for Lisa, 52. 'My dad is 90, my mum is 83. I have three kids. Everyone wants a piece of me and at the end of the day there isn't enough left for me! Oh my God, my greatest joy is to sit with a good book and a decent coffee. I don't suffer fools any more. I'm no longer intimidated by health professionals or by people in authority. I choose to surround myself with people who help lift my life state up, not down. I'm fiercely loyal. I have no time for people that use or abuse my help. I prefer quality over quantity – and that goes for wine, coffee and people.'

'Self-care is important to me,' agrees June, 'and since last summer I have made more of an effort to focus on it. I have picked my moisturising rituals as my easy route to self-care. They relax me and only take a few minutes each day but make a big difference. Self-care can feel like another obligation, and so my view is, start with something really small that you enjoy and make that your self-care ritual.'

Lots of women I spoke to raved about American author Gretchen Rubin's book *The Four Tendencies*. Self-help books make me shudder but, as more than one person said it had cured them of their people-pleasing, I bought it and did the 'Which tendency are you?' test. (I love a test.) It wasn't hard. In a nutshell, the four tendencies are: Upholder, Questioner, Obliger, Rebel. They're pretty self-explanatory TBH. And even though I am 99.99 per cent sure I am much better than I used to be at disagreeing, confronting (where necessary) and saying I want a curry if I want a curry, I still recognised myself instantly as an Obliger. (Maybe with Rebel rising.) And, as the word implies, being an Obliger is not flattering. It is the word that sums up the most people-pleasing of people-pleasers. People who are good at doing what other people want, being motivated by external indicators and rubbish at paying attention to their own. They are the people who can't write a book without a deadline hanging over them (that would be me), the people who can only go running when they've signed up for a marathon, the people who will cook a meal for someone else but not for themselves. 'People who will exhaust themselves meeting obligations for others – feel burned out and also resentful because they don't meet their expectations of themselves,' says Rubin. Ugh. They are absolutely bloody rubbish at self-care and often 'can't find time for it'. Oh dear oh dear oh dear. In my defence, I'm on it.

The nadir of this behaviour is the secret longing to get sick. Something I used to identify with to a mortifying extent. Three times in my life I have been wiped out by illness. With the benefit of hindsight, I can see now that it was burnout or a breakdown; on each occasion the illness was my body's way of saying enough, because I couldn't be relied on to do it myself. Once, while I was at university, in a toxic relationship I really, really needed to get out of, I was struck down by gastric flu, had to be taken home because my flatmates were too worried to have me around, and missed the end of term. Once when I was editor of *Cosmo*, I had an infestation of mouth ulcers so bad I could eat nothing but ice cream (could be worse) and when I phoned the doctor to ask when I could go back to work, the duty nurse screamed at me that I was 'not that bloody important'. Not the best bedside manner, but she wasn't wrong. And again, towards the end of *Red*, when I was chronically anaemic and kept passing out in the street, instead of going to bed and staying there to nurse the bruises on my face, I insisted on going to Milan for the shows. I got a chest infection that became bronchitis that became pneumonia with a little added MRSA. In each case, it was as if, my mind unable or unwilling to make the decision to sign itself off, my body had to take over. Every time those illnesses came, much as they took me out for over a month in each case, inside, all I secretly, shamefully, felt was immense relief.

It turns out that illness – proper no-choice-but-to-take-to-your-bed ill, but not life-threateningly so – is a real fantasy for many women. I *do* know how terrible that sounds and I obviously don't mean to make light of serious illness. (Especially since I write this in a climate of Covid-19 lockdowns.) I just mean ill enough to have to take a compulsory month out, somewhere no one can make demands of you. To be signed off from life, from responsibilities and obligations. If you like.

'That really resonates with me,' Genevieve said. 'Although my husband is a shite carer when I am really sick so I would need to be hospitalised to get a proper rest! However, I have on a number of occasions said to both [him and my son], "I resign from my position of mother to this family." So yes – with the benefit of age and wisdom – I'm trying not to take this any more and this year will be trying to do more for me!'

'I know exactly what you mean,' says Joy, who has recently been treated for an aggressive form of breast cancer. 'When my sister and I were young, my mum used to wish out loud for tonsillitis so she could justifiably take to her bed. Even when I was chronically ill, I longed for the anaesthetic of major surgery to step back from coping with cancer and fighting for life: to take a break from keeping everything together for us all. I felt the only

187

way to really rest was to spend a week in hospital. That's shocking and sad and unnecessary. But I've emerged determined to take up more space, take more time, look after myself as I expect others to do. That said, I don't see my husband needing an anaesthetic to escape! Men don't have me-time. They just live in the space they have, in the time it takes.'

Then she tells me a brilliant anecdote. One that is so resonant I want to get it made into a poster and plaster it all over social media. 'Once, in our very early twenties, my best friend and I were in a café on Brighton seafront,' she wrote. 'We saw a man our age stretched out on a wall, arms above his head, shirt off, asleep in the sun. We marvelled at his ease in the world. He just stretched to take as much space as it took. Twenty-five years later we still refer to him as the boy on the wall. Escape and connection and responsibility and stretching to take up space, those things are all key to me.'

To me, too. I truly believe there's something about menopause that encourages – or forces – us to take those things for our own. To do what has been socialised out of us and take up space; put our own needs front and centre. Or maybe it's that and experience; by the time you're this old you know that the cliché *what doesn't kill you makes you stronger* is a cliché because it's true. And, you know what other cliché is also true? *You can't please all of the people all of the time.* So, you know, you might as well please one of them, and why shouldn't that one be you? That could take any form. It could simply mean applying moisturiser, as it does for Paula, or going for a run every morning. It could be bigger. It could be lying on the wall taking up all the space you need.

Recently my husband and I made a big, life-changing decision. The decision to restart our lives at the other end of the country. In another country, in fact. By the time you read this we will probably be there. That decision came at the end of an extremely tough few years. After a low to end all lows. Everything had

changed. Professionally, emotionally, financially, you name it. It
became important for us to take a long hard look at our lives and
be honest with ourselves and each other about what we needed.
What we *wanted*. We wanted to take the sow's ear of the previous
five years and try to turn it into a silk purse. We're going back to a
place that has always mattered to us. A place where, in Jon's
words, we decided that there was an *us*.

We didn't make the decision lightly, we didn't make it without
considering the other people it might affect – our family, our
friends, our work obligations – but we thought long and hard, and
we made it. It's the right decision for us. We're happy with it. Half-
excited, half-terrified. Everyone else? Not so much. We are, in fact,
surrounded by people who think we're doing the wrong thing and
have spent a lot of the last year telling us why. And, painful as that
is, that's OK. I can hardly believe I typed that. I'm going to type it
again. That's OK. It is. It's OK. Other people are not happy. They
are angry, they are cross, they are upset, they are sad. They are
allowed to be. And yes, I feel bad that they feel bad because of
something we're planning to do. And that's OK, too. Because for
almost the first time in my life I feel that I'm allowed to do what I
need to do and they're allowed to have feelings, too. After a lifetime
of trying to stop other people feeling bad, it's a revelation.

Taking up space physically and emotionally is a big learning
curve. I wasn't brought up like the boy on the wall. Not many
girls are, no matter how hard their parents might try. But I'm
learning to Be More Boy On The Wall, at least in some aspects of
my life. Going with my gut. Doing what I think is right. Doing
what makes me happy. I still give a lot of fucks, more than I'd like
to but fewer than I did. I'm getting better but it's slow progress.
To suddenly be comfortable with who you are after decades of,
well, not being. To speak up for yourself and stand your ground.
To stop worrying about what everyone thinks all of the time isn't
going to happen overnight. But it's coming. And I like it.

'This is such a crazy time in a woman's life hormonally. It's a whole different ballgame, a thrilling and terrifying trip. Everyone tells you the lights are starting to fade but it's like, no, you still have so much beautiful life yet.'

Kathryn Hahn

12

THE SEXUAL SHIFT AND THE MID-LIFE SPLIT

What happens to our sexuality once babies are
no longer the order of the day. Why some women
shift, some split and some soldier on

'I don't fancy men any more,' says my friend Liz. I raise my
eyebrows, curious to see what's coming next. Is this a precursor to
'I'm leaving Marc'? Or is this just a general comment on the state
of her personal nation?

We're sitting in an over-priced wine bar around the corner
from her office. In true central London style, its over-pricedness
is making zero difference to its popularity and, despite it not yet
being 6pm, it's rammed with the post-work for-God's-sake-give-
me-a-drink crowd. A table was out of the question and we're
perched at (not literally ON the bar, I'm assuming...) the corner of
the bar making short work of a bottle of whatever dry white wine
is second on the wine list. We're both drinking too much, too fast,
on empty stomachs (the token 'we better eat something' olives are
sluicing around somewhere in the wine) and within 20 minutes
we're suddenly talking – much too loud, because that's the only
way we can hear – about sex, in a way I haven't since I was about
17. I can't remember where it came from as two minutes ago we

were talking about her crap boss and how if she had to spend one more day smiling sweetly while he mansplained her own ideas back to her she was going to tell him where to stick it. I suppose there's a kind of alcohol-fuelled logic to it, as she's just been telling me how much she loathes one particular man and the surrounding men who suck up to him.

'I fancy women,' she elaborates and tops up our glasses as she reels off a list of famous-ish women who, to put it bluntly, she *would*. The list is topped and tailed by Phoebe Waller-Bridge.

I get it. Now I think about it, I *would*, too. (In the unlikely event that you're reading this, Phoebe, sorry if that's more information than you bargained on.) And Kristin Scott-Thomas's *Fleabag* character. And Megan Rapinoe. And Winona Ryder. And Keanu ... But then, if you're a member of the Gen-X female population, there's always Keanu. I'll admit fiftysomething me finds fiftysomething Keanu hotter than ever. So hot, in fact, that I've even sat through *Destination Wedding*. Anyway, Keanu diversion aside, when I start to think about it I'm surprised to find I can drum up quite the list.

'Women are just so much more interesting,' Liz continues as, for some unknown reason, we signal to the barman for two glasses of Fino. It's nice. Dry and not very sherry-like. 'I'd rather spend an evening hanging out with my funny smart female friends than any of the men I know. Except Marc, obviously.'

I've never met the father of her children, but I assume he's nice, smart, funny, because she is and so are their kids. Then I think about my other female friends; both long-standing friends and recent acquaintances. They are almost uniformly smart, funny, interesting, interested. And, incidentally, predominantly but not exclusively straight, with relatively long-term partners. Almost all, if I hazard a guess, not hugely interested in men for men's sake. Unless they too are smart, funny, interesting and interested; then it's a different story. It makes me wonder how much of a difference gender makes. Liz and I ponder this, made philosophical by our second glass of Fino. We are both 50ish, both menopausal (within seconds of grabbing stools, we discarded our blazers – regulation uniform of the menopausal 'still got it' – and too much wine isn't helping the overheating situation. I already know I will regret this tomorrow. And the next day.) Both heterosexual up until this point. Possibly *just because*.

On the tube home I look around the carriage and think about that old tube ad that went: 'One in three people on the tube is attractive, so if one of the people on either side of you is hot, it isn't you.' It was snappier than that, of course, but that's the gist. I glance furtively either side. So far so good. Then I scan my bit of the carriage. Then I look further down. By this point I've forgotten the rule of three because what's struck me is this: none of the men are hot. Or even remotely interesting-looking. In fact, they leave me absolutely cold. I'm sure the feeling is mutual. I'm a middle-aged woman after all, plus I'm a bit pissed and it's not even 9pm. I'm not under any illusions. But in the light of my conversation with Liz it seems significant, because sitting there on the Northern Line I can't remember the last time I encountered a man in the course of my everyday life that I was actively physically attracted to. It could be the kind of men I tend to meet: with a few honourable exceptions the lovely, warm, funny ones are invariably gay or my friend's husbands or my husband's friends; the rest are aggressively performatively masculine – and often working in finance, advertising or sales. They might well be funny, clever and interesting – who knows? – if they stopped willy-waving long enough for anyone to find out. (I guess some people find that attractive, but it always just made me want to chop it off.) It could also be, of course, that I'm not looking, because I'm not.

But it's not that, because, now I think about it, where women are concerned it's a different matter. I work across industries overflowing with smart successful women. Until I started working from home I met women with great taste and bags of personal style every day of the week. I have coveted their bags, their hair, their unattainably expensive Bottega Veneta shoes. Barely a week passes without me crushing on some high-achieving woman's style on Instagram. (This week it's the *FT*'s Jo Ellison. Next week, who knows?) I've lost count of the number of times I've interviewed a woman and thought how I would love to go for a drink with her, spend more time with her, have a laugh and a chat, get to know her. When I interviewed Cheryl Strayed, we joked about going on a bar crawl at two o'clock in the afternoon, mainly for the walking and talking in between bars. The killjoy film publicist wasn't having any of it. I have met many women in the last decade with whom I have struck up lasting – if not live-in-their-pockets – friendships. I care what they think. I'm interested in their opinions. I love spending time with them. When I think about it, almost the only other person that applies to is my husband. I can, I realise, absolutely see how you might get here – on the other side of kids (if you have them), menopause, social expediency – and think fuck it, I'm much more interested in spending all night talking to her than listening to X snore.

There is plenty of evidence that desire – sexual or indeed otherwise – is dynamic and mutable regardless of age. Particularly if you're female. In *Sexual Fluidity: Understanding Women's Love And Desire*, Lisa Diamond, PhD, professor of developmental and health psychology at the University of Utah, describes sexual fluidity as 'situation-dependent flexibility in women's sexual responsiveness'. She goes on to explain: 'This flexibility makes it possible for some women to experience desires for either men or women under certain circumstances, regardless of their overall sexual orientation. In other words, though women – like men – appear to be born with distinct sexual orientations, these orientations do not provide the last word on their sexual attractions and experiences. Instead, women of all orientations may experience variation in their erotic and affectional feelings as they encounter different situations, relationships, and life stages.'

Diamond is no random scientific outlier. She has been researching sexual fluidity for more than two decades and, slowly but surely, society is coming around to her way of thinking.

'We're not talking about bisexuality, when someone is attracted to both genders at any given time,' says Sheryl Kingsberg, former president of the North American Menopause Society, who hosted Diamond's research at their annual conference in Philadelphia in 2017. 'Aside from orientation, there's also the concept of sexual fluidity – that women can, at one point, be completely in love with a man and then at another point be completely in love with a woman. And that can change once or that can change several times throughout her life. It's not that these women have been closeted lesbians their whole life, or have been in denial about their true feelings. These are women who were perfectly happy with men and are suddenly seeing and feeling things differently.'[28]

But there's something else interesting going on here. In 2010, Diamond made this comment to the *Guardian*: 'In my study, what I often found was that women who may have always thought that other women were beautiful and attractive would, at some point later in life, actually fall in love with a woman, and that experience vaulted those attractions from something minor to something hugely significant.'

Think about the implications of that for a moment. Who hasn't stopped to admire another woman's shoes, hair, style, sense of humour, way with words. Who hasn't had a girl crush (horrible phrase, sorry) on another woman at work for one or several of the above reasons? That's not to say that every time we admire another woman we're taking a step on the road to sexual fluidity – although, so what if it was? It simply means that women have long built bonds with other women, regardless of who they conduct their sexual relationships with and, for many, our girl-friends are at least as important as our boyfriends. In short, if you have always been inclined to appreciate women, to build meaningful relationships with them, Diamond posits, you are more likely to fall for one as you get older.

This is a point first made by the poet Adrienne Rich in her 1980 essay 'Compulsory Heterosexuality and Lesbian Existence'.[29] It's long and complicated and fascinating, but what it boils down to is that the denial of women's sexuality (you know how lesbianism was never illegal because Queen Victoria wouldn't have it that women did that sort of thing?) is a means to control and suppress any transition, creativeness and economic advancement of women. Regardless of the efforts of male-dominated societies to channel us into 'heterosexual reproduction', Rich argued, women regardless of history and culture 'always managed to form intimate emotionally primary ties to other women.'

And those ties can sometimes be life-saving. As Harriet, 48, who recently separated from her husband of 24 years, says, 'The thing that has really sustained me through this time is my girl-friends. We joke that if we could take a gay pill we would because it would make life so much easier.'

What's stopping you? I ask. 'In theory I could see that happening,' she says and then laughs, as if making a shameful admission, 'but I really like men! I really like maleness. And I've never met a woman who made me feel I could totally turn for her. If I did I'd be delighted.'

I put this theory to several of the women in my email group. The split was about 50:50 between those who spat out their tea and those for whom it ignited a flash of recognition. But even among those who dismissed it out of hand there was undeniable wistfulness; a definite romanticising sense of 'I wish'.

Women who discover same-sex feelings later in life have been dubbed 'late-blooming lesbians'. Of course. Wherever there's a journalist there's a catchy alliteration, but I'm not sure it's an entirely accurate description of what's happening here. It sounds too ... definite. Too, intentional. Too 'right at the lights', when it's probably more like, 'ooh, that road over there looks interesting'. Combine that with the fact that the generations below us – millennials, yes, but far more so Gen Z – are embracing pansexuality (in a recent YouGov poll, more than 50 per cent of 18–24-year-olds described themselves as something other than 100 per cent heterosexual) and increasing numbers of women in the public eye are taking a look at that more interesting road and signalling back that, oh shit, yes, it *is* interesting, come and have a look. Like branding guru Mary Portas, now 60, who had two children with her husband of 14 years, before marrying and having a son with fashion journalist Melanie Rickey. Or bestselling novelist Elizabeth Gilbert, now 50, who left her second husband José Nunes (the Love bit of *Eat Pray Love*) to live with and love her best friend Rayya Elias through the cancer that killed her in 2017. Or actress Cynthia Nixon, now 54, who was married 15 years before falling in love and having a son with Christine Marinoni in 2004. Or musician Alison Goldfrapp, now 54, who has been with her first female partner Lisa Gunning for ten years. Or bestselling children's author Jacqueline Wilson, 70, who has been with her partner Trish since her marriage broke down in her early fifties.

I don't know about you, but I believe we fall in love with people not penises. It just so happens that for me, so far, the person I fell in love with happens to have one. In Diamond's seminal study, around a quarter of the women reported gender was largely irrelevant in their choice of sexual partners. 'Deep down,' said one woman, 'it's just a matter of who I meet and fall in love with, and it's not their body, it's something behind the eyes.'

It is, isn't it? When I met Jon, I fancied him, yes, but it was his brain, his quirky world view, his questioning approach to life, his values, his taste in books, all these things and more that I fell in love with. And that goes for most of my friends, too. Alison Goldfrapp is the same. In 2010 she told *The Sunday Times*: 'I think of everything as being about a person and a relationship, and I am in a wonderful relationship with a wonderful person. It just happens to be with a lady ...'

Mary Portas said the same of her relationship with Melanie Rickey. 'In one way it was just about Melanie. But there was a sexual attraction. I do love women.' After they split, after 17 years together, she told *The Times*: 'I've been in love with two men and one woman. What does that make me?' Fluid, that's what. And the fact that both Portas and Gilbert appear to have since embarked on relationships with men (Portas – ever the PR maestro – teasing it in an interview, Gilbert announcing her love for British photographer Simon MacArthur, a friend of Rayya's, on Instagram) doesn't imply some sort of error, it simply confirms that for them sexual attraction is about the person not their gender

I have always felt I'd have wanted Jon whether he was male or female; and I don't think I'm speaking out of turn when I say I'm pretty sure the same goes for him. After all, when we played the fantasy hall-pass game, we both chose Johnny Depp. (Yes, I know, but that was before he left Vanessa Paradis and we all discovered what he was like.) I think in another iteration, we both chose Tilda Swinton.

Lisa Ekus, 61, was married twice and had two daughters before she met her partner Virginia Willis 15 years ago. 'Although I'd always appreciated the wisdom and friendship of other women, I never thought I was gay,' she told the *Mail on Sunday*'s *You* magazine. 'I believe it is who Virginia is as an individual that attracted me to her. My comfort level with this woman is far greater than I have ever felt with the men in my life. Virginia is not only wonderful and smart, but she meets my intellectual and emotional needs.'

It's a view echoed by bestselling author of *Untamed* Glennon Doyle, who, aged 40, left her husband of 14 years to be with former US soccer player Abby Wambach. 'When Abby walked into that room, I actually felt the words *there she is*. This was just an absolute recognising of the person I was supposed to be with for ever.'

Freya Blom tells a slightly different story of falling in love with a woman after 16 years of marriage to a man. 'I never thought of myself as fluid in my sexuality. But I always believed, and still do, that people should "never say never", she writes in a blog for The Gottman Institute. 'The truth of that belief came crashing into my consciousness when ... I realised I was falling in love with someone else – and was shocked and amazed to find that that someone else was a woman. I can remember first meeting her and thinking she was great, and that I had the beginnings of a new best friend ... As I followed that intuition and we interacted more, I realised it was more like a best-friendship on steroids. Super-charged, powerful, and magical ...'

What if menopause is that magic combustible ingredient that throws everything up in the air and just wanders off, leaving you to see where everything lands and either pick up the pieces or roll in the hay? Not a million miles from adolescence. Except you're kind of prepared for adolescence (kind of ...) and not trained to deny its very existence. Unlike menopause.

In an interview with Lotte Jeffs in *You* magazine, Diamond suggests it could be ... 'What we know about adult development suggests that people become more expansive in a number of ways as they get older ... I think a lot of women, late in life, when they're no longer worried about raising the kids, and when they're looking back on their marriage and how satisfying it is, find an opportunity to take a second look at what they want and feel like ... Puberty involves a heck of a lot of change, but you don't choose it. There are life-course transitions that are beyond our control.'

Think about the chaos puberty causes. What if menopause is that plus experience? Anything could happen!

Diamond also cites research by psychologists Celia Kitzinger and Sue Wilkinson. In the mid-nineties, they interviewed a range of women who undertook abrupt transitions from heterosexuality to lesbianism in mid-/late adulthood. Their conclusion? 'They are no more driven by biology or subconscious urges than they are when, for instance, they change jobs; such choices could be viewed as influenced by a mixture of personal re-evaluation, practical necessity, political values, chance and opportunity.'

It makes sense to me. All around me I see women in their late forties, fifties and beyond, suddenly putting their heads above the parapet and asking themselves 'is this it?' Then, depending on 'personal re-evaluation, practical necessity, chance and opportunity', doing something about it. That something doesn't necessarily involve another woman. It could just as easily be deciding to upend your life for another man or simply for yourself. But it usually does involve a dramatic shift of some description and most often on the relationship front. A 'mid-life epiphany', to steal a rather brilliant phrase from Lisa Ekus, that can manifest in myriad different ways that all have one thing in common: domestic upheaval.

When I ask my email group about their relationships – how they feel about their partners, their sex lives, their level of satisfaction – I'm met largely with silence. It's only when I email a second time suggesting I may have struck a chord that the answers come, first trickling, and then flooding, in. And the picture is not that pretty. More than half were either dissatisfied in their relationship or had already left it. Many relatively recently. Their reasons were as diverse as the women, but few boiled down to the boredom of having been in a relationship with the same person for, in some cases, more than 20 years. In the main, if these women left for anyone, it was for themselves. Perhaps because they've finally reached a point in their lives when they can put themselves first.

This was certainly the case for Harriet. 'My counsellor told me that at this age men leave for other women, and women leave for themselves. Because they just can't bear it any more. It's weird, the number of people among my peers who are certain I must be having an affair with someone else to have left. There's a really pervasive view that to be this age and a woman you must be seeking security. It's like, who would want *you* at this age? Why would you give up a relationship that provided you with security to be out there on your own? That's such an old-fashioned, sexist view. I left for me. Because I had to, for my own sanity.'

'I see this a lot,' says June, 46. 'Some of my girlfriends feel it's a critical time for their relationship. It's stick or twist. Many have chosen to twist, as they just don't want to settle or grow old with their partner. Kids have left and they have nothing to talk about any more. Those on the other side are happier in the longer run and many aren't looking for a new partner. I don't think it's any coincidence that this is timed with the second phase of life that's the menopause.'

Of course, not everyone leaves, not everyone wants to, but just as many are sitting there wondering *what if.* Stephanie, 49, met her husband when she was 17. They've been together ever since. 'So ... here we are,' she says, rolling her eyes. 'Still together. But *woah* have I wanted to walk away numerous times in the past five or six years. We've had the odd rough patch, no more or less than anyone else in a long-term relationship, but I totally get why women want to leave for themselves and not someone else.

'My husband isn't a bad egg, he's a good dad and he's kind, but he's also a typical beer-swilling bloke who wants to get pissed with his mates every week and I'm bored of it. I constantly wonder "Is this it?" And I worry we will have sod-all in common by the time we retire. This year I'm pushing myself (and him) to do other stuff outside of our comfort zones, but Jesus it's hard work because he can't be arsed. Bless him for wanting a simple life – a shag, two bottles of wine, Kung Po prawns and golf most days, stopping off for three pints on the way home – but that's *his* dream life. It's not mine.'

201

Kate Spicer, who split with her partner of ten years at the end of last year, totally identifies with the 'fix it' mentality many women apply to heterosexual relationships. 'Women will try to fix things and in fixing themselves they hope they'll fix someone else, but men don't do that fixing work on themselves. I wanted to have some couples therapy just to educate ourselves about each other, look at bad patterns we'd got into, but he was like "no, no no". Men become really conservative with a small c. They're conservative and they're frightened – afraid of outsiders, germs, change ... Men are like Republicans, women are Democrats. The vagina is just a more liberal kind of space!'

Kate describes the break-ups 'sweeping through' her social network. 'Everybody's coming up to 50. They're all dealing with men who haven't changed. They don't move. They're like a train shunted into a siding and that's where they stay. One – she's gorgeous and she's married to someone famous – and when I talk about the "stuckness", she's like, "Yep, it's doing my fucking head in and I don't want to stay." She's got everything. He's clever, he's funny, he's rich, he adores her. But he's not going to fucking change.'

Kate has a point. Many men don't change. They don't have to, it's not integral to their very existence the way it is to women's. From puberty onwards we change day to day, week to week, month to month, and then, at the end of it we have 'The Change'. And we have no choice but to change again. Our bodies are constantly in flux. As Diamond said, 'Puberty involves a heck of a lot of change, but you don't choose it. There are life-course transitions that are beyond our control.'

We are changing and we are looking outward for new experiences. As Harriet put it, 'When my kids left home I got a release of energy. I wanted to be out there. Feeling things, exploring, feeling mentally free at last. I think, at that point, a lot of men don't feel like that. They don't need to. Lots of women I know around my age are seeking to push outward and expand their horizons, if they can afford to.'

For Rowena, 54, like Harriet, 'pushing outwards' signalled the end of her relationship. 'I do believe (peri)menopause was a contributory factor to my marriage disintegrating,' she said. 'I "suddenly" felt I wanted a bigger, bolder life. It was like a lightbulb went on and I was roused from a long (pleasant) slumber. Not many people could understand this. I had a perfectly nice life with a very nice, decent and handsome man. They were either "jealous" or resentful because my actions shed a light on their own often less-than-happy-and-fulfilling marriages/partnerships.'

More than one woman I spoke to reported feeling 'a surge' of anger. Something had to give. Or else. Whether their personal shifts were sexual or relationship focused, it was not a choice but an imperative. There was no way back. Only forward. Fix it or ... fuck off out of it.

'When the hardcore parenting years were over it felt as if, suddenly, I had time to reflect on how I felt about my own life and future,' says Caroline, 55. 'It was as if I'd lost my gumption during the parenting years and had fallen into an almost subservient and certainly compliant role ... We were close to breaking up. My husband didn't want us to – and my terms for staying together were: getting a cleaner, selling our home and moving to a city flat. We did all that and weathered the storm. Five years later, we are probably closer than we've been since our early days, pre-children.'

But a surprising number of women choose not to fix it. They've had enough. For those women, 'fucking off out of it' was scary but exhilarating. 'It's frightening if you've been in a long-term relationship, to be out there and have people only see you as a bunch of crow's feet and greying hair is slightly anxiety making,' admits Harriet. 'There was a period where I fully felt I'd never have sex with anybody again. Also after two decades of having sex with the same person, the idea of taking your clothes off in front of someone new is daunting. In fact, everyone I know who's done it has done it drunk!

'When I was in my twenties, sex was very much tied up with emotion and power balances and complex sexual politics and the thing that has surprised me this time around is that I *can* separate sex from emotion, in a way that I certainly couldn't when I was younger. I really surprised myself by saying, after one fairly nice kiss, "do you want to come back to mine?", which still makes me laugh at the thought of it. He was more nervous than I was. I'd got myself into a terrible anxiety – has everything changed in the last two decades: does everybody want anal and not expect anyone to have pubic hair? The joy of sleeping with someone the same age is that they feel the same. It was all fairly traditional, like riding a bike, it turns out.'

Rowena agrees. 'For the last three years I have had a lively dating life. Initially I felt like a kid in a candy shop ... all these cute men who wanted to spend time with me. (And not one of them over 40!) It was fun and exciting to feel so wanted. A great ego boost. It made me feel alive.

'Sex is much more fun and fulfilling,' she goes on. 'In no small measure because I know my own body so much better than I did in my twenties and thirties. I know what I want and feel confident asking for it.'

For Jenny, 48, divorcing her partner of 27 years felt like 'being stuck in a stuffy room where there's no air and someone just bashed open a window and I was able to finally gulp in the air and breathe. It was wonderful. I'm now craving experiences and the sisterhood. At this moment I couldn't care less if I never saw another cock again. I was married to one for long enough! All I want to do is strengthen the female friendships I have let slip and find new ones as I venture out and hopefully find other like-minded women.'

Jenny also had another, even more significant, motivation. 'It wasn't just the growing awareness of approaching 50 and thinking, "I cannot live the same amount of time feeling like this." My daughter was 14, and it dawned on me: "I am a shit role model. I am colluding with this man over his behaviour. I am staying bound and small and frightened of rocking the boat." All the things that, if I saw my daughter repeating them, I'd want to scream FUCK THAT! YOU ARE WORTH SO MUCH MORE THAN THIS! And one evening, something so small and innocuous happened and I heard a discernible voice inside of me saying quietly, but urgently, *Enough. I'm done.* And I went to the solicitor's the next day.'

'I decided to quit using my daughter as an excuse not to be brave and start seeing her as my reason to be brave,' writes Glennon Doyle in *Untamed.* 'I would leave her father and I would claim friendship-and-fire love, or I would be alone. But I would never again be alone in a relationship and pretend that was love.'

Her point? Teaching our daughters their lot is to be martyred for their own children is a bad bad bad bad look. As Doyle says, 'What if a mother's responsibility is not showing her daughter how to slowly die? What if a mother's responsibility is showing her daughter how to fight to live?'

The way society programmes us to accept some hypothetical heteronormative lot is insidious. Women have long been socialized to believe that providing and receiving emotional support is part and parcel of a relationship, a duty, or an obligation. Anticipating, reading and responding to our partner's emotional and physical needs is ingrained.

So ingrained that even if we think we're not having any of that patriarchal nonsense, the truth is we often are. Writing in the *New York Times*, Stephanie Coontz, author of *Marriage, a History*, looked at the differing division of emotional labour in heterosexual, gay and lesbian relationships. She examined three fascinating and disturbing studies. In a shock to no one it was the women in heterosexual relationships who fared worst.[30]

In the first study, carried out in 2019, researchers asked three sets of legally married couples – heterosexual, gay and lesbian – to keep daily diaries recording their experiences of marital strain and distress.[31] Women in different-sex marriages reported the highest levels of psychological distress. Men in same-sex marriages reported the lowest. Men married to women and women married to women were in the middle, recording similar levels of distress. 'What's striking,' says the lead author of the study, Michael Garcia, 'is that earlier research had concluded that women in general were likely to report the most relationship distress. But it turns out that's only women married to men.'

An earlier study in 2006 'found that the happiest and most sexually satisfied couples are now those who divide housework and childcare the most equally. Couples where the wife does the bulk of routine chores, such as dishwashing, report the highest levels of discord.'[32] Further, a 1999 study found that when a never-married man married, he reduced his routine housework, on average, by three and a half hours a week. When a woman married, she *increased* her routine housework – the numbing work that must be done each day – by almost that much.[33]

Add to this the findings of a massive 2018 study that found that heterosexual women have fewer orgasms than any other sexual demographic – and substantially fewer than heterosexual men – and you can't really be surprised we're starting to shift![34] But you can when you think none of this applies to you. Only to turn around and find that, 'Oh, it does'. And it's that moment. That, *oh, it does*, moment that leads many women to walk.

'I think men want to be looked after, especially as they get older,' says Lisa, 52. 'They may well have been reasonably independent in their thirties but ultimately, as they approach 50, onwards, they don't want to face the twilight years alone. You know what, neither do I. This is when I look at my partner of 16 years who stimulated my mind with endless debates and whom I found knowledgeable on the most bizarre subjects and I think, I'm well and truly fucked!'

'About five years ago I became conscious of all the unpaid work I did in the home,' says Deborah Campbell, 49. 'I got very angry about it (hormone-fuelled) and began to speak differently about the work in the house. I started talking about it as work that needed to get done for the house to function and for all of us to benefit. The work was not for me, I needed nothing doing. It didn't change overnight but it has changed. I would say it's more or less 50/50 now.'

'Have you ever heard a man talk about "me-time"?' asks Lena, 56. 'Yet women do constantly.'

She's right. Most men don't need me-time. When I look around at the women I know in roughly my age group, most of them have spent years compromising themselves – what they want, who they are, their jobs – and more and more are reaching a point where they've had enough. This is particularly true of women with children. With some exceptions, I've watched women's lives be transformed by having children, while the men's have carried on more or less regardless. As Lena put it, 'Men have a career and happen to have kids. Women have kids and happen to have a career.' There is no research to back this up, just ask any woman in the street with children in tow.

Andrea Hewitt, founder of the blog A Late Life Lesbian Love Story, came out at 40 when she had two kids. Isolated and with nowhere to turn, she started her blog. She was clearly on to something because its private Facebook group now has 1,800 members. They have one common thread, says Hewitt, and that's having put their own lives on a back burner when they had children. 'I'd say a lot of the people in my group have a very similar personality type. We're mothers, we're fixers, we're problem-solvers; we want to focus on everything but ourselves. It isn't until you have time to do some self-reflection that you go: "Wait a minute, what about me?"'[35]

That 'what about me?' moment, a mid-life epiphany, a sexual/gender shift. Whatever you call it, whatever you choose to do with this new surge of energy/fury/outward burst into the unknown, we now live in a world that is decidedly different from the one we grew up in – a world that, in many ways, feels less judgemental of people who choose to live life their own way than it used to. I grew up in small-town Hampshire in the 1970s, a world where 'lezzer' and 'homo' were the playground's favourite insults – especially if, like me, you weren't a girly girl. My eighties puberty wasn't much better. Girls who lost their virginity were slags, sluts and whores. Girls who didn't were frigid.

But the world is different now. And thank God for that. Partly because millennials and Gen Zers won't put up with that shit, they won't suffer periods and mental health problems, racism, sexual harassment and impending environmental doom in silence. Partly because equal marriage is in the statute books and Harvey Weinstein is in prison; and partly because more and more of us have been brought up – and have brought our own daughters up – not to sacrifice themselves on the altar of femininity. Which is handy, because there's a fair chance you're about to have a bit less of it! Or at least a different, less traditionally feminine kind of it. TBH I identify with eighties model and musician Leslie Winer, who says, 'Performing femininity was not on my list of things I thought I'd be good at.' Me neither, Leslie. Me neither.

In truth, I always found 'presenting as feminine' (as opposed to female) a pain in the arse, but I appreciate that's not the same for everyone. I'd like to look good (as opposed to good for my age) and I still have hair that comes halfway down my back. But whether you have long hair or short, go grey or keep dyeing, exercise your body into submission or accept those extra inches, chances are you're going to feel and look, well, a bit less like a girl. And I say that as someone who takes HRT, so don't tell me it's entirely the oestrogen because it isn't. It's not included in any of the symptom lists I've found – and God knows there are hundreds of them (symptoms, and lists) – but at the same time, feeling less feminine is something that crops up again and again in conversation. Not everyone likes it. Some see it as a release, others as a failure. It's partly internal, but maybe it's also external.

Maybe, just maybe, some of us can no longer be bothered. Or you could put it more proactively and say that maybe we are just redefining our femininity in a way that makes us feel more comfortable.

'Without hormones my femininity is fraying,' says Darcey Steinke in *Flash Count Diary*. 'Twice I've been called Sir. Once by a parking lot attendant and a second time by the young man who bagged my groceries. I did not correct them. Instead I tried to sit with the idea I'd been misgendered. I don't possess the strong female signifiers I once did. My hair is not long and shiny, my skin is no longer smooth. Plus I do less to support my gender artificially. I wear more androgynous clothing and rarely put on makeup. I've lost interest in "doing" my female gender, propping it up.' Like me, Steinke admits, she feels more comfortable in her new body, her new persona, her jeans and her boots. Much less so on the rare occasions she has to dress like a girl. 'When I do dress up for a wedding or a bat mitzvah, I feel like a drag queen, performing a gender out of sync with my physicality; but unlike a drag queen, I don't feel that gender is natural or correct.'

Perhaps what we're talking about here, post-menopause, is not so much a sexual shift as a gender shift. You can see it as shifting forwards into a new age of putting yourself first, or you could see it as almost a shifting back, ever so slightly, to our pre-adolescent selves. The selves who put themselves at the centre of their entire existence. The selves who, in the words of Nora Ephron, aspired to be the 'heroine of their own lives, not the victims'. Perhaps now we can decide who we are and what we like because we like it, not because society tells us we should. It's an opportunity to harness new experience, with fewer boundaries. A new lease of life, if you like. A new lease of sexual life.

You might be happy in your existing relationship, you might want to have a relationship with a woman, you might want a relationship (or several) with another man. You might not want to have a relationship at all. And that's fine. That's your decision, to live the next phase of your life your own way. What strikes me, though, is how many women no longer want commitment of any kind. For some it's an active choice, for others it's because they had it and found it suffocating; a case of once bitten twice shy, and no way are they going anywhere near Tinder. Each to their own. All that matters is we own it.

Harriet, after 20+ years of marriage and three kids, just wants a fuck buddy: 'A happy time and some laughs and some good sex and to feel comfortable. If I can find someone who does that, I'm happy, I just want to feel like a sexual being.'

For Sarah, 69, who describes her romantic life as having been, 'So many relationships, so little love and commitment – on both sides, sometimes,' has chosen to be on her own, after four children and three serious long-term relationships, the last of which was with an alcoholic. 'There are a few evenings when it's just me and a book or the TV and, for a few minutes, I feel lonely. But it doesn't last. I have chosen to be on my own rather than risk another relationship.'

For Jenny, 'The thought of having sex for fun and being liber-ated I think is brilliant and I so admire women who are doing that ... But I have no idea what I really like sex wise. When Gary Lineker said he wasn't massively into sex, he liked the flirting side of things and that was that[36], I remember thinking, that is *exactly* me! I love the fun of chatting to men and a bit of a connection.'

Newly single, Kate Spicer is tentatively exhilarated. Actually, scrap the tentative. 'I haven't felt sexy for a while. I've had sex and I've had good sex but I haven't felt sexy. It's more ... having a bit of sass, a bit of swagger. It's so weird that this break-up is happening, so obviously a lot is changing in my life but I feel sexually interesting again – I don't know if that's the hormones or being single. The whole prospect of being a 50-year-old single woman ... it sounds awful, but because I don't feel weighed down by it, I think it will be fun.'

'While some people find change threatening,' Diamond told the *Guardian*, 'others find it exciting and liberating, and I definitely think that for women in middle adulthood and late life, they might be the most likely to find sexual shifts empowering ... I think the notion that your sexuality can undergo these really exciting, expansive possibilities at a stage when most people assume that women are no longer sexually interesting and are just shutting down, is potentially a really liberating notion.'

But it's her last point that fills me with hope – excitement, even – for women who are shifting, opening up the potential to move on from the people and things that might have limited them in the past. 'Your sexual future might actually be pretty dynamic and exciting,' she says, 'and whatever went on in your past might not be the best predictor at all of what your future has in store.'

'Women have been given an extension. We were brought up to think that by this age it would be all over, but it doesn't feel like that any more. It's not as awful as I thought it was going to be.'

Frances Barber

13

HOW TO BE WHAT
YOU CAN'T SEE

*The ignored percentage, because when did
you last see a woman who looked like you – in
a magazine, on the internet, on TV?*

The morning I sat down to write this chapter, Billie Eilish said this: *'Some people hate what I wear, some people praise it. Some people use it to shame others, some people use it to shame me. But I feel you watching, always. And nothing I do goes unseen. So while I feel your stares, your disapproval or your sighs of relief, if I lived by them, I'd never be able to move. Would you like me to be smaller? Weaker? Softer? Taller? Would you like me to be quiet? Do my shoulders provoke you? Does my chest? Am I my stomach? My hips? The body I was born with, is it not what you wanted? If I wear more, if I wear less, who decides what that makes me? What that means? Is my value based only on your perception? Or is your opinion of me not my responsibility?'*

As nothing is real unless it's on Instagram, I posted it on Instagram, pulling out the quote: *The body I was born with, is it not what you wanted?* 'She's such an incredible role model for our children,' someone commented immediately. 'And for me!' I joked back. But I wasn't joking. Billie Eilish may be an 18-year-old girl struggling with an 18-year-old girl's issues (albeit with a rock star's bank account and a mind-blowing quantity of talent and drive) but she's a shitload more sorted than I have ever been, and her statement spoke directly to me. It went straight to the heart of the contradictory place in which I have found myself these past few years: confounded and discomfited by the divergent expectations imposed on women no longer of 'childbearing years' and, until recently, lacking the self-confidence to tell those expectations to do one.

The expectations demand one of the following: 1) Look 20 years younger. And keep looking 20 years younger till the day you die. Or 2) Shuffle off into your dotage to seek serenity with your dog and your sensible shoes and don't bother us important people going about the busy work of making the world go round. Oh, I forgot there's another option. 3) Be the butt of the joke, because that's the only time most people will pay any attention to you. Think white men dressed up as middle-aged women – or more accurately old bags – a la *Mrs Brown's Boys* or embarrassing overstuffed middle-aged sitcom women having a hot flush while all the other characters mock her.

How about none of the above?

We all need role models. No matter how self-contained we think we are, or might appear to other people, most of us need someone to look up to and if that someone looks like us, walks like us, talks like us, so much the better. And if they don't – which they usually don't, especially not when you're a woman north of 50 – then we take our role models where we can find them. Hence the popularity of Eilish and her fuck-you anthems amongst the peri- and post-menopausal women I know.

Role models are a complicated business for 'older women' (as a side note, try googling 'older women' and see what you get. Google, it turns out, cannot tell the difference between 'older' and 'elderly'. Stairlift, anyone?). But you can times that by a thousand thousands if you're a woman of colour, differently abled, working class, LGBTQ+ or any combination of the above. I'm a middle-aged, heterosexual, white Western woman from a working-class background living a middle-class life. There ain't no way anyone straight and white – even if they are female – is under-represented. But! Nevertheless, with diversity at the heart of almost every conversation, I'm here to say that ageing is the unsexiest diversity there is and so I am going to write a chapter on how to be what you can't see when you're a woman north of 50.

Think about it. Women over 45 make up almost 46 per cent of the female population in the UK alone, and 52 per cent of the total population over 45.[37] We have time, disposable income, experience on our side. (The third of the UK population that's over 55 now accounts for 47 per cent of consumer spending.) All things that could make a huge difference to businesses that are currently struggling to keep afloat in the face of digital onslaught, economic chaos and global pandemics. If only they bothered to represent us. The media seems to have forgotten we exist (unless certain elements are slagging us off for paying either too much attention to our appearance or not enough). I'm not sure the advertising industry ever knew we existed (certainly that's how it feels to us, according to a study by JWT that found that 72 per cent of American women over 50 don't believe advertising applies to them. The Women's Worth study by UM London found that 46 per cent of women in peri- or post-menopause say they aren't represented by advertising and 44 per cent feel patronised by it), which I guess is hardly surprising since about 100 per cent of adverting decisions are made by men. (I'm exaggerating, but only slightly.) This starts to make a sick sort of sense if you get an insider take on the way the industry (notorious for 'ageing out' both men and women but particularly women) operates. In a piece for shots.net, self-confessed 'pain in the arse' Amy Kean (also brand and innovation director at the agency &us and author of the hilarious *The Little Girl Who Gave Zero Fucks*) puts it like this: 'The ad industry is riddled with crap audience definitions ...

Even now, most audience definitions begin with age. Age is a planning comfort blanket. This lazy, un-insightful proxy for likely-to-purchase. And immediate – also lazy – assumptions are made by planners upon hearing an age. Assumptions about life stage, lifestyle and outlook on life.'

She goes on: 'In the media world, over 35 is old. Apparently I woke up on my 35th birthday a cougar! With no libido. Grey, matted hair and lacking lust for life. I started going to the opera and feeling sad. On the day I turned 35 I stopped having periods, leaked while running for the bus and began dancing really badly. I became Conservative. Shunned high heels and sought comfy shoes (actually that last part is true). Target audience definitions are a joke.' When I stopped laughing I felt a bit sick. It would be funny if it wasn't so horribly, bleakly, infuriatingly true.

And as for the fashion industry, don't get me started. True, it occasionally dabbles with older models, but as we've seen they tend to be very old, very thin, very quirky or ideally all three. Usually enlisted for publicity stunts rather than actual inclusivity. As Lyn Slater, @AccidentalIcon, put it after she and Alyson Walsh (That's Not My Age) were dubbed InstaGrandmas in a feature in *Elle Japan* and lumped into a category encompassing women aged 50–80, 'This is the only way I am ever written about any more. I feel erased as an individual; not empowered … Everything else about me except for my age is now deemed unimportant or insignificant. In the guise of addressing ageism, my multiple social positions, achievements, history, and uniqueness are discounted, leaving me feeling ever more invisible. This is fetishising age; not admiring it.'[38] This fling usually lasts a season at most, before the diversity baton is passed on to race or differently-abledness or body positivity. The beauty industry is marginally better, but only because it knows it can sell us stuff so we can pretend to the rest of the world we are not – whisper it – getting older.

When I was writing the pitch for *The Shift*, I spent some time analysing the representation of older – let's say 45 upwards

– women across the media and advertising. (I say 'analysing', I mean I read some magazines and watched some telly.) The impression I was left with was that women like me didn't actually make one. I read a range of glossy magazines that were approximately 40–50 per cent advertising and found that, on average, women over 45 featured in two ads, both of which were for beauty products. Yep. Two. Out of more than 300 pages. That's some marginal representation. (And, of course, both those women were white. And one was Helen Mirren. I love her but, really, you'd think we'd moved past the rule of 'we've got one, we don't need another one' by now.) Editorially, there were no women over 45 in their pages with the exception of one feature about older women doing amazing things, like having careers ...

Then I turned my attention to TV. By which I mean the kind of TV you get if you turn on the box in the corner of the living room of an evening (not Netflix or Amazon Prime or Apple). I know hardly anyone under 40 does this any more, but I still find it strangely comforting to flick aimlessly through dozens of channels and find nothing very interesting to watch. In the course of a full evening – approximately six hours – there were ... drumroll ... four. Sue Barker, Fiona Bruce, Emily Maitlis and Cathy Newman. All excellent women, I'm sure, but hardly representative of an entire demographic or even a fraction of it. Of course there are others who just didn't happen to be on that night (Kirsty Wark, Clare Balding, Gabby Logan, Kirstie Allsopp, Mary Beard ... so far, so white). And to be fair, I could get that number up a bit by dropping the threshold to 40, but why should I make it easy for them when they don't make it easy for us?

Just in case the situation had radically improved in the last seven or eight months I decided to repeat this exercise yesterday. (Procrasti-researching.) And you know what? It had. A bit. In the April 2020 issues of the glossies I analysed, there were not only four ads featuring women over 45 – and one of those ads featured four women, three of whom were over 45! Yes, yes, one of those women was Helen Mirren, but one of them was a woman of colour, Denise Lewis, 45. Titchy witchy baby steps. But steps nonetheless. It gets better. While 'older women' are only really allowed to advertise skincare – when they're allowed out at all – they are also allowed to flog us fragrance. Stand up Julia Roberts, 52, for Lancome (for now let's overlook the fact the brand famously ditched Isabella Rossellini for being 40 because they've been paying for that little error for decades now) and Cate Blanchett, 50, for Armani. But I've saved the best for last because the door that has always been closed to us insufficiently skinny, quirky old birds is fashion. You will never ever see a woman over 30 advertising fashion unless they're making a thing of it and hoping to get some publicity – Joan Didion in Celine sunnies, for example. Or they're advertising embarrassing mum clothes that no mum I've ever met has been seen dead in since the 1950s. Less than 2 per cent of models were Gen X in spring/summer 2018 fashion campaigns.[39] But lo and behold, just as I was about to give up, there, on the inside back cover of *Vogue* (and believe it or not, that's a prestige slot, not somewhere you bung an ad if it's a bit embarrassing and you don't want anyone to see it), was Charlotte Rampling, looking stunningly androgynous and wrinkled and lived in and glorious in Givenchy. Of course, Rampling is borderline Didion territory but let us have this little moment of joy.

(And then, as if that wasn't enough excitement for one year, British *Vogue* went and really spoiled us by putting Judi Dench, 85, on their June cover.)

Could this transformation be replicated on the box? Miracle of miracles, it could! First of all, there was the woman presenting the local news (BBC South if you're interested), then there was Sandi Toksvig, 61, Pru Leith, 80, and Jenny Eclair, 59, on *Bake Off*, Joanna Lumley, 73, and Miriam Margolyes, 78, on competing primetime travelogue programmes. (I can't honestly say I look at any of them and think 'that's me', but how can you not love

Margolyes, a woman who happily admits to sitting on people who don't give her their seat on a train – that was pre-Covid-19, of course.) But then I perked up because there was also *The Split*, starring five – FIVE – women over 45. Don't tell anyone, they might make it stop. And if you really cheat, which I did, *Mrs Fletcher* – the adaptation of the Tom Perrotta book about a middle-aged woman and her teenage son's respective sexual awakenings starring Kathryn Hahn, 46 – was on Sky. Not remotely intersectional, admittedly, but better.

Had something shifted, or was it a fluke? Or was it, perhaps, a reaction to the improvements forced on the movie industry by #MeToo, #TimesUp, #OscarsSoWhite and #OscarsSoMale and, of course, by the inexorable rise of the streaming services, not to mention a bunch of gobby middle-aged women on social media yelling that they'd had e-bloody-nough of being ignored.

It's not even ten years since Cher was quoted as saying, 'In my job, becoming old and becoming extinct are one and the same thing,' the 40-year-old actress Julie Hoang sued website IMDB for revealing her age on the grounds that this would wreck her chances of working in an industry where 'youth is king', and you could count the actresses still working past their mid-late forties on one hand, if not one finger. So there is no way you can say we haven't made progress. Now I can reel off a list of actresses on both sides of the Atlantic making a healthy living: Cate Blanchett, Julianne Moore, Juliette Binoche, Olivia Colman, Sharon Horgan, Sandra Oh, Viola Davis, Tina Fey, Julianna Margulies, Laura Dern, Kerry Washington, Naomi Watts, Salma Hayek, Amy Adams, Tracee Ellis Ross, Sandra Bullock, Nicole Kidman, Helena Bonham Carter, Emma Thompson, Kristin Scott Thomas, Helen McCrory, Tilda Swinton, Lena Headey, Fiona Shaw, Sally Hawkins, Taraji P. Henson, Siobhan Finneran, Sarah Lancashire, Helen McCrory ... Truly that is off the top of my head and I'm sure I've missed hundreds more.

My personal favourite though is Keeley Hawes, 44, who has gone from sidekick and support to best character ever in *Line Of Duty* and leading two of last year's greatest TV hits, *Bodyguard* and *The Durrells* (on which she, quite literally, ran the show). 'Historically you're not supposed to be getting to my age and having the time of your life,' she said in a recent interview. 'But the parts are getting much more interesting ... I'm no longer apologetic. It doesn't all end in your forties. There are lots of us.'

She's right, there are. 'When I turned 50, I worried it was downhill all the way,' Helena Bonham Carter told *Harper's Bazaar*. 'But it's been quite the opposite. I don't think I've ever been happier or more fulfilled. This huge blooming of television means character-driven stories, so there's a lot of choice and a lot of work. When I was young, you were considered "older" over 30.'

This is in no small part because women are taking control of the means of production quite literally: screenwriters Sally Wainwright, Sharon Horgan, Sarah Phelps, Emma Thompson, Phoebe Waller-Bridge, Jojo Moyes and Andrea Gibb, among many others, writing incredible, identifiable, *real* roles for women; producers like Alison Owen (*Suffragette, How To Build A Girl*), Sally Woodward Gentle (*Killing Eve*), Ceci Dempsey and Lee Magiday (*The Favourite*), putting women's stories front and centre. Not older women specifically, just women per se. And, of course, there's Reese Witherspoon. She's not everyone's cup of tea but Witherspoon has to get a large part of the credit for driving change in Hollywood.

'How wonderful it is that our careers today can go beyond 40 years old. Twenty years ago we were pretty washed up by this stage in our lives. That's not the case any more. We've proven ... that we are potent and powerful and viable. I just beg that the industry stays behind us as our stories are finally being told. It's only the beginning,' said Nicole Kidman, one of the happy recipients of Witherspoon's activist energies. I would agree with Kidman on everything here except for the begging bit. Take a leaf out of Witherspoon's book and don't beg, *demand*. If you don't like the way things are being done, make like Witherspoon and get on and do it for yourself. And Witherspoon didn't like the way women's stories were being told in Hollywood. Or more crucially, weren't being told at all. 'It was getting laughable how bad the parts were, particularly for women over 35,' she told *Fast Company*. 'And that, of course, is when you become really interesting as a woman.'

She spoke to 20 studios and only one was developing something with a woman in the lead. 'I felt a responsibility to my daughter and all the women in the world to create more opportunities for women,' she told *Glamour* magazine. 'We're 50 per cent of the population.'

Of course, those roles are for actresses of all ages, but the upshot has been that, as Kidman put it, actresses who would previously have been 'washed up' at 40 aren't quite so washed up any more.

Think about some of the biggest hits on both the big and small screen of the last few years and Witherspoon and her production companies have been responsible for quite a few of them – first Pacific Standard, the company she launched with Bruna Papandrea that made Cheryl Strayed's *Wild* and Gillian Flynn's *Gone Girl*, and now Hello Sunshine, which she has self-funded with a minimal injection from venture capital to such stratospheric levels of success that she has no need to let Hollywood studios invest in her movies. Instead she has projects in the works for Hulu, Apple and Netflix. In the last couple of years, Hello Sunshine has been responsible for *Big Little Lies* – three of the five lead actresses (Witherspoon, Kidman and Laura Dern) having a combined age of 146; *The Morning Show*, on which Jennifer Aniston – the latest of Hollywood's newly anointed fabulous fifties – put in an award-winning turn; and now Celeste Ng's *Little Fires Everywhere*, starring Witherspoon herself and Kerry Washington, 43. Along the way Witherspoon has reignited careers – most notably her own (the woman's not a saint), but also those of many of the actresses she works with (Dern in particular has become hot property) and the female authors she champions with her book club. Strayed, Ng and many others have benefited. The message here is not that what Witherspoon is doing is either philanthropic or perfect – there's no denying that, with the exception of *Little Fires Everywhere*, she is almost exclusively telling white women's stories and using white actors – it's that if you want something doing, maybe you just have to do it yourself.

Witherspoon and co have made leaps and bounds; they're role models for sure but they're still unattainable every which way you look at it. Which brings me to Jennifer Lopez. Who knew one 50-year-old woman's body could be quite so divisive. It started when she wore *that* Versace dress on the catwalk in 2019. She had made the lauded but not rewarded *Hustlers* the same year and, it has to be said, was in smoking-hot shape. That appearance in that dress went some way to winning her ad campaigns for Versace and Coach. I thought she looked pretty fabulous. And frankly, from where I'm sitting, a 50-year-old woman fronting a fashion campaign is a 50-year-old woman fronting a fashion campaign. Yes, J-Lo's body brings new meaning to the word unattainable, but then it always did. Whether I'm 20, 30, 40 or 180 I'm never going to have J-Lo's booty. Nor am I prepared to put in the hard slog to get it. Then came Super Bowl. Oh lordy. J-Lo and Shakira – combined age 93 – shaking it up in sequins in the Super Bowl ad break is the best thing I have ever – or will ever – see. For the duration of their performance they owned that stadium; they looked like they were loving every minute and every woman I know over 40 wanted some of it.

'Seeing Shakira, a 43-year-old woman, having the time of her life playing the drums in her golden suit made me so happy,' said Anna Carey on Instagram. Lucy Brazier agreed: 'I messaged my peri-meno friends and said, "Watch it! Ignore the overtly sexy stuff, just revel in the power and joy. They are not 20."'

Rowena and Paula also thought J-Lo and Shakira were fabulous. 'Whether or not their bodies are unattainable didn't cross my mind. Personally I believe it's inspiring rather than depressing or intimidating to see "older" women who look amazing,' said Rowena. 'To be honest I was blown away by J-Lo and Shakira,' Paula added. 'OK, I will never and have never looked like them but at 50 next month myself *cries gently into my cashmere cardigan and wrings out my Tena Lady* seeing them smash it makes me strive to keep working that bit harder.'

Then came the incredulity bordering on outrage. On Twitter a meme began trending comparing Rue McClanahan, aged 51, when she took on the role of Golden Girl Blanche in 1985, with J-Lo aged 50 in 2020. How could this be? How could this woman be 50? What was a 50-year-old woman even doing at the Super Bowl? Let alone performing at half time? Who let her out? The astonishment was both understandable and really bloody insulting. (As Buzzfeed's senior editor Rachel Wilkerson Miller brilliantly tweeted, 'perhaps we should let women over the age of 40 do things more often.') Yes, J-Lo does look incredible. She looks incredible for anyone at any age. She's an actress. She's a singer. She's a dancer. She's a *performer*. She pole dances like a bastard – and that takes serious core strength, it's no wonder she's got those muscles. Plus she's loaded. It is her job to look incredible and I don't doubt she invests a shedload of time and money making sure she does. (While the rest of us are drinking wine and watching Netflix.) But it's a job that she does really, really well. Let's hear it for her.

But this is not 'what 50 looks like' any more than it was when, 40 years ago, Gloria Steinem famously retorted 'this is what 40 looks like' when told she didn't look her age by a reporter. Well, yes and no. She's right, in that 40 then bore zero resemblance to 40 two decades earlier, and nor does 50 now bear any resemblance to 50 two decades ago. Fifty looks as many different ways as there are women. And while few of us look like our mums and even less like our grandmas did at 50, 50 seldom looks like J-Lo. Or, for that matter, Jennifer Aniston. It's just that we rarely see anyone who doesn't. This undeniable fact left plenty of people raging.

'Great she's there, great she's redefining what you are "allowed" to do at 50, but why does she look like she did at 35?' says presenter and diversity activist Grace Woodward, 44. 'It's still peddling the same narrative of as long as you successfully achieve sexy and hot you still get let in. As long as you look young, you're still relevant. I'm not sure it's helping me move into my fifties with confidence at all ... I hope I won't still be having to trot out the heels and tits to have good sex and be valued at 50. It just makes me feel sad.' Sad, and exhausted, according to Nahid, 52. 'She looks amazing, of course she does. She's J-Lo. However, doesn't it just bring up the possibility that we're going to be expected to look bloody amazing till the day we die?! How tiring ...'

'I'm quite happy with the J-Los and Shakiras and all the other unattainable beauty standards being out there and showcased, because what they're doing is continuing to do what they do and continuing to be who they are,' says Susie, 47. 'That's one of the things I've struggled with more than looks. What – because I'm 47 I'm suddenly meant to behave and look a certain way!? Nope, it's not for me. I'm not about to don my slippers and sit knitting with a cup of tea (though I do love all three and rather love them together) ... I'm being me and I'm quite happy that I'm seeing people out there who are more representative of me than the images of older women we used to have.'

Which brings me back to that infuriatingly ageist and sexist reaction after the Super Bowl, not just to J-Lo's fabulousness but to how incredibly good she is at her job, at 50. It enrages me to have to put those two things in one sentence, as if we don't expect 50-year-olds ... no, let me rephrase that ... 50-year-old *women* to be good at their jobs. It's a point writer Ayelet Waldman made in an interview with Next Avenue. 'I had a professional situation where someone – an elderly man – actually called into question my abilities both as a woman and as a menopausal woman. Now, I'm not menopausal yet, first of all. But I will be soon, really soon. And to hear him saying that was horrifying. He's worked throughout this period of his life, many decades past where I am now, and I'm sure he would have been horrified at the thought that anybody would have called his capacities into question at age 50. I'm sure he felt vital and at the prime of his life, right? But somehow, there was a question whether I could do the work ... I had no idea that as soon as I got to this age, to be a 50-year-old woman, the sexism gets completely complicated by this idea that not only are you incompetent as a woman, but you're incompetent because you've reached your senescence! Or something.' The situation was complicated further by the fact Waldman's husband – the writer Michel Chabon – just 18 months her senior, was not having this issue at all. 'In their eyes he's still young and vital,' she added. Strange that.

Truth is, there is no issue with J-Lo being fabulous. The real problem arises when J-Lo being fabulous, being J-Lo, is the only image of a fiftysomething woman living a public life we get to see. And right now it is a dominant image. So much so that when we do see a woman in her late forties looking like a woman in her late forties, we go slightly nuts. That's what happened to Californian artist Alexandra Grant – 46, super-chic, 'embracing her grey'. Of course it wasn't helped by the fact she had the temerity to be on the red carpet holding hands with the internet's favourite boyfriend, Keanu Reeves (famous man, 55, dates woman in the vaguest vicinity of his own age. Shock horror.). Grant, of course, is cool, interesting and successful in her own right, exactly the kind of role model I had in mind when I started this chapter, but whatever. Who cares about that? Just as the internet was patting itself on the back for its gender- and age-inclusiveness, it went and spoiled it when, a few weeks later,

Reeves took his mother, costume designer Patricia Taylor, 76, as his date to the 92nd annual Oscars. Within minutes she was being mistaken for Grant. Well, you know, they both have grey hair. They're both 'older' women. Who cares if there's 30 years between them ...?

'Do I feel represented at 52? Hmmm, let me see ...' says Lisa. 'Why, yes, by adverts for bladder incontinence, over 50s life insurance and Saga holidays. Perhaps the occasional token Hollywood actress advertising L'Oréal skincare.' (There's Helen Mirren again ...)

'I feel that I am not really represented anywhere, to be honest,' says Clare, 48. 'All the women I see who are meant to be me – as in my age and experience – white middle-class heterosexual women, are always beautifully dressed, fantastically made up, and just seem so together. I feel wholly inadequate compared to them.

'Even when you see ad campaigns that are meant to represent all women, like Dove, you never see disabled women, women who actually wear glasses, women who I look at and think – that's me! All the time we are bombarded with images of women who are so far from reality that it's just disheartening.'

'I think we often muddle representation with realism,' says Louise Nicolson, author of *The Entrepreneurial Myth*. 'We are still represented by Shakira or Sue Barker, even if their bodies and brains remain completely unrealistic from our own personal perspective. The only person really like me, is me. If I'm enough as I am, which I think I am, I can shrink those fabulous women on screen and just enjoy them for capturing a relatable emotion or moment. Forget literal imitation. Seeing J-Lo in full flight was glorious but we all have sequin-dress-at-the-Super-Bowl moments if we make it our business to notice them. Mine include dancing in the early hours at my friends' wedding or a run on a bright blue winter morning. Unremarkable, unrepresented, totally missable moments by all but me. We need to look around us to understand the potential of being our age, in this age. We'll miss the moment waiting for the media to catch us up and represent us in our full variety. I think you can be what you can't see in the media – as long as we are seen by those who matter most.'

Ourselves, and women like us. Look around you at the real women you know. The women you admire and look up to – in life, in your family, in your workplace and, yes, on Instagram and on TV. When I asked my email group, the names that came back were as varied as the women who came up with them. They ranged from Marian Keyes to Joan Bakewell to Carine Roitfeld to Isabelle Huppert, Amy Poehler, Shonda Rhimes, Zoe Ball, Claudia Winkleman, Monica Bellucci, Toni Collette, Maya Rudolph, Oprah, Hermione Norris, Fay Ripley, Brigitte Bardot, Diane Keaton, Ruth Bader Ginsberg, Jane Garvey, Fi Glover, Jamie Lee Curtis, Katty Kay and Geena Davis, plus an endless list of female friends and family.

But this is not just about us, middle-aged women sweating it out in the here and now. This is about younger women, too, all colours and classes and gender identifications. Writing on Refinery 29, Sara Raphael summed up the extent of the problem. 'I'm only 31 and I already feel aged out of things, already feel "older", less desirable, past my prime … I want to be at my most stylish, my most confident, my most powerful and desirable. I want to look forward to those years, not spend lots of money and emotional energy trying to stave them off.' She's right. If I had seen older women as a matter of course – doing things, being things, going about their daily lives – would I have felt quite this rudderless for the last few years? Quite this ambivalent about claiming and championing my age and experience? For young women to even begin to start to imagine a different sort of life as they mature, we need to see ourselves, the 40, 50, 60, 70-year-old woman, represented in all walks of life. Otherwise it's not just us who have nothing to aspire to, it's the women coming after us and the women coming after them.

Imagine a world in which young women can't wait to be 40, 50, 60 and beyond. I know it sounds like a sick, sad joke from where we're sitting but it doesn't have to be. We can change it. Because, let's face it, no one else is going to. And we can make a start right here by standing up for ourselves and other women, speaking up and voting with our feet, our mouths and our wallets. And if you're reading this thinking, nobody cares what I think, I have two things to say: 1. You're wrong. Don't write your-self off just because you think society does. (And yes, I know there are plenty of days when that is far easier said than done.) And 2. If you really believe that, then why not show your support for other women who are doing it for you right now instead?

Women like Cindy Gallop, the ad industry irritant, who stops at nothing to call out sexism and ageism in the ad industry and beyond. Bernardine Evaristo, whose sheer tenacity saw her make history at 60 as the first black woman to win the Booker Prize. The take-me-or-leave-me common sense of psychotherapist Philippa Perry, the outspoken front of Jodi Picoult, the open-heartedness and truth-living of Elizabeth Gilbert, the sheer Cheryl Strayedness of Cheryl Strayed. Marian Keyes for being Marian Keyes and endlessly ramming home hard messages in between the gags. And I love the fact that the biggest literary events of the past year have been Margaret Atwood, 80, and Hilary Mantel, 67. Oh, and Neneh Cherry, just because she's Neneh Cherry. (She's so cool!) And Patti Smith. More in and of herself than anyone else I can think of. And Tilda Swinton, mainly because she's taken on Alan Rickman's mantle of go-to Brit whenever Hollywood is looking for a baddie. And Scotland's First Minister Nicola Sturgeon. And New Zealand premier Jacinda Ardern. And all the other female world leaders who dealt calmly and intelligently and decisively with the Covid-19 pandemic while many of their male counterparts ... didn't. And, yes, I admire Reese Witherspoon, several years my junior, for quite literally seizing the means of production.

These women are all in their way role models. I could go on and on and on. But every single one of them has something we all have if we look inside ourselves – they have the energy, they have the couldn't give a fuckness of being interesting and interested, grown up, just a little bit over it. And that doesn't mean that they or we don't give any fucks, it means they try to only give the fucks that matter.

Follow them. Cheer for them. Champion them. Because that's the only way to make change.

'The best way to look at ageing is to see it as an opportunity to leave what didn't work behind and step boldly into a brand-new future.'

Oprah

14

WITCHES GET SHIT DONE

Aggressive, difficult, bossy? You bet. Why it's time
to stop putting up with macho shit at work

It's what feels like day 935 of Fundraising Round Two and, yet
again, my partner-in-pitch-purgatory, Jo, and I are the only
women in the room. We're not fazed by it, a little bored certainly:
by now we are entirely used to pitching The Pool, which is barely
months old and has got off to a flying start, to various groups of
men (predominantly white, predominantly middle-aged,
predominantly so alarmed to find themselves talking to women
over 30 that they don't know what to do with their body
language) who don't really have a clue, or any interest in, what
we're talking about. We have our routine down by now. Our pitch
deck has been fine-tuned to within an inch of its life and our
patter is always broadly the same: Jo opens, I do the creative
vision, the need we meet, the response we've had, the users who
are already saying they didn't know what they did on their daily
commute before The Pool existed, the brands who've already
given us cold hard cash (they usually perk up at that point), and
then we share the future strategy, the opportunity, and Jo does
the numbers. We vary it a bit according to the audience – some
potential investors are experts in the media landscape, others not
so much; some are interested in the international opportunity,

others just want a spreadsheet – and the degree of boredom in their expressions, covert and not-so-covert smartphone swiping and curveball questions. All of which, to be honest, is better than silence.

This particular presentation is to a lone middle-aged white man in a Savile Row suit. (And I've seen some immaculate, very much not-off-the-peg suits since we started raising money. Investors tend to either look like they've just stepped off Savile Row or like they never stopped wishing they were one of the Beastie Boys. There doesn't seem to be anything in between.) This one would definitely consider himself a silver fox. And, frankly, given the size of the private equity fund he manages, he's probably justified in feeling he can consider himself anything he wants, because the chequebook is in his hand. We get to the end and he asks a couple of desultory questions. Not bad, but definitely not good either.

'It's not really my sort of thing so I sent it to my wife,' he says. Here we go. 'And she sent it to some of her friends ...' We wait. Listen to the traffic four floors below. The same exhaustion and frustration I feel is emanating from Jo. Groundhog pitch. Another half an hour of our lives we won't get back, but we swore to 'have every coffee' since it was one such coffee that led to our founding investors (a couple – the female half of which had adored Lauren's radio show and *Red* when I edited it), and so every coffee is what we have. But the way these pitches are going, it should be 'kiss every frog'. This is legit a frog. 'They liked it,' he says, smiling benignly, like he's giving us a little present. 'But they had some suggestions. If we proceed we will want to discuss them.'

This is not the first time – nor will it be the last – that we have been presented with 'wives' suggestions'. It has been made very clear to us since we started raising investment that The Pool is 'a girl thing' and the investment pool, being more than 80 per cent male, is not hugely interested (not unless we're planning to expand into ecommerce because they can get their head around flogging people stuff). And so we often find ourselves batted over to wives, girlfriends and the very occasional female investor. This is one such time. As well as a wife and her friends, he has one female investor who may (heavy on the *may*) be interested. He'll get back to us. I've heard this before. Dozens of times. It means no. In my, by now extensive, experience, an out-and-out no would be better because we wouldn't spend the next week refreshing our email.

Then he leans forward with a patronising smile on his face. 'Can I give you some advice?' He doesn't wait for a response because we don't get to say 'No ta'. The advice is coming, like it or not. 'Next time,' he says. And like a tragic little puppy dog desperate for approval my heart leaps. There will be a next time! 'Bring a man. You girls don't do a bad job, but it would lend you some gravitas and make the investors feel more comfortable to know there's a man involved.'

We nod, push back our chairs, shake hands, put on our coats and wait in silence for the lift. I think we may even have thanked him for his time. It's only once we're back on the street that the shock morphs into fury. Bring a man?! What the actual fuck?! I want to run back upstairs and punch him.

The girls in question were 48 (me) and 46 (Jo). Together we had almost 50 years' experience at the top of the British magazine industry and between us had made many millions of pounds for the companies we'd worked for. With The Pool's co-founder Lauren Laverne, we'd just launched a digital platform for women that was punching way above its weight, putting the wind up some of the industry's biggest names, with nothing more than half a million pounds (which looks like a lot written down but is sod-all for a media launch (UK *Glamour*'s launch marketing budget was £5 million, *Grazia*'s rumoured to be an eye-watering £12 million – and don't get me started on how much *Vice* and Buzzfeed burned through), sheer bloody-minded determination, a healthy social media following and insane levels of hard work from everyone on our small team. But regardless. *Bring a man if you want to be taken seriously.*

I'd like to say that was a one-off. It wasn't. There was the private investor who 'didn't see who would use it' because he – a fiftysomething white man – wouldn't. (In fact, there were dozens of those.) There was the venture capitalist whose specialism was 'the space where media meets tech' (I know) who told us to add 'fairy dust'. 'You mean bullshit,' I said. He shrugged. 'Call it what you like.' The unspoken? I don't care what you call it, you'll add it if you want my money. We didn't add it. We didn't get his money.

And there was the potential investor who'd already made a fortune from a blink-and-you'll-miss-it social media unicorn, who told us that 'if [we'd] added a nought [he] would have invested'. We didn't add a nought – because we knew we couldn't deliver that extra nought – and no, he didn't invest.

By the time we actually encounter a female VC, I'm ashamed to say I assume she's someone's assistant. In my defence that's because she not only opens the door herself but offers to make us coffee, not something that has ever happened in a VC's office before. Which tells you pretty much everything you need to know about women at work. When she comes into the room carrying a tray, heels the door shut behind her and sits down, I have to stop myself doing a double take. 'I've been here six months,' she says. She's fully engaged and asks the most switched-on questions we've had so far. 'And you're the first female founders I've seen.' 'Same here,' we mutter.

'Did you think ...?' Jo asks, when we get out of the meeting. I nod and hang my head in shame at my unconscious bias against my own gender. The unconscious bias I would have sworn I didn't have before I started spending most of my waking hours in finance and tech land.

But worse even than being told that investors would only feel comfortable with us 'girls' if we brought a man along was the

American techbro who'd made a fortune on start-ups before his 25th birthday. He sat across the boardroom table from Jo, Lauren and me, late one Tuesday afternoon at the end of a board meeting, looked us in the eye and said, 'I think you have a great product here and it's got some potential, but I'm worried you ladies will get tired. You're not so young any more.' I still don't know how none of us punched him. Lauren was only in her mid-late thirties. But he showed not the slightest hesitation or flicker of embarrassment. Like almost every other techbro I met in the five years I worked on The Pool, his ego was unconstrained and his confidence commensurate with his bank balance. It didn't occur to him that whatever he thought might a) not be correct or b) be better off not coming out of his mouth. I guess since he probably couldn't even see 30 in the distance by squinting, I, at 48, was inconceivably old. Certainly old enough to be his mother. So how I was still walking unaided, let alone starting a business from the back of a napkin in Pret, he probably couldn't begin to imagine. They don't say investors invest in their own image for nothing. (Hence all the money that goes to white men. Here's one of my favourite fun facts, just to keep you entertained: in 2019 more VC-dollars were invested in WeWork than were invested in all female-fronted businesses put together. Softbank poured $5 billion into WeWork (and lost it). That's $1.5 billion more than the total VC investment in all female-founded companies in America in the same period.[40]) But there I go, making excuses for men at work instead of calling them out. I've been doing it ever since I got my first job. It's time to stop.

Ask yourself, how long have you been putting up with macho shit at work? Colluding with it, covering it up, dumbing it down as if it's all a joke and, well, boys will be boys and they just can't help themselves, and maybe it was your imagination or you're overreacting or you can't take a joke. Or putting up with it because you feel grateful just to be there? As a working-class comprehensive-educated kid who didn't know what public school

was until I went to university, the only thing I knew about
Oxbridge was that the brainiest girl in our sixth form had been
rejected, even though she got straight As (although chances are
that wasn't just a class or gender issue but a race one, too ...).
Then I got to London and every other person I met had been to
one or both. I lucked into a job on a magazine, and that was how
I felt: lucky, like I'd fluked into someone else's life. I was a gobby
22-year-old with a lot of front hiding the fact I had no confidence. Plus zero understanding of office politics. I soon learnt.
Underneath I was terrified that someone would realise they'd
made a mistake – that the interviewer who rejected me from the
periodical journalism course at the London College of Printing
when I was 17 had been right when he said I 'didn't have what it
took to make it in journalism' – and I'd get kicked out. I was so
grateful to be there. And, even when I was running some of the
country's biggest magazines, and people told me I was the scary
one, I couldn't quite believe it. How could I be scary when I was
terrified?

You might work in a female-dominated industry that's run by
men, like I did. You might work in a male-dominated industry.
Or you might work for yourself. But whichever industry you work
in, I bet you too have spent a fair proportion of your working life
being mansplained, manterrupted, manspread and manhandled.
I have been shouted at, ignored, been told to bloody do what I
was bloody told, had the table fist-slammed by a male CEO for
not agreeing to something. I've had my ideas stolen, been
endlessly talked over. Like every other woman I know I have had
my own thoughts explained back to me 24 hours later by some
man who thinks he's a genius. I have been asked to make the tea,
take the minutes, and pop out for loo roll. And all of those even
more so when I was running my own business – a business I
co-founded, in part, to get away from the men dominating the
industry in which I had spent my working life ... In those five
years I made more tea, took more minutes, tried to bite my

tongue at more bouts of willy-waving and bought more milk and loo roll than I had in the previous twenty-five. Oh, the irony.

I thought the corporate media landscape was bad. And, yes, it is sexist and ageist, no doubt about it. (Also classist and racist ...) But it was in start-up land that I learnt the really harsh lessons that I wish I'd learnt decades earlier. And I was taught them by two groups of people: 1. middle-aged white men – it didn't matter whether I worked for them or they worked for me, they still treated me like the help. Maybe that's an exaggeration but, on the whole, they certainly didn't treat me like an equal. I finally – too late to save the business – learnt the cost of letting them. And

2. millennial women – the young women who worked at The Pool – weren't having any of it. Not from men. Not from their peers. Not from their bosses. Not from me. I found them astonishing and terrifying in equal measure. In the main, though, I admired them for their utter self-belief and conviction. I remember when #MeToo first happened, I tried to explain how it used to be, starting out in your career in the late eighties, early nineties. During one news conference I told them about a men's magazine staffer who 'everyone' knew could not be trusted around female interns. When it came to a head, did he get reprimanded? A written warning? Fired? Nope. Nothing. But the management did take action. They stopped hiring female interns. I always knew it was horrifying. I was simply illustrating the climate in which Gen-X women had started work. The young women I was relaying this to were disgusted, not just because of the blatant abuse of power but because of how we responded. And they had a point. It *was* disgusting and if 'everyone' knew, why did no one do something? They were right. *Someone* should have. And that someone should have been me. Or any one of the other women in vaguely senior positions who'd heard about it on the company grapevine. Easy perhaps to say from a privileged 21st-century perspective. Substantially less easy back then to actually do. It was a lesson, though. One of many I learnt working with those young women. They weren't brought up by women who'd had to put up and shut

up, and who had taught them to do the same, they were brought up by us. Many of the younger ones had mums roughly my age. The battles we fought and lost back then weren't their concern. The mistake I, and many other Gen-X women, have always made was to believe we had to play men at their own game. We thought we had to, we thought we should be grateful to have a seat at the table, even if we were expected to keep getting up from it to pour the tea. But when you play people at their own game, you lose. It's *their game*. Duh.

Jenny, 48, acknowledges that she spent far too long doing precisely this. 'I backed down, I stroked their ego. I found ways of making them feel something was their idea. I showed other women how to do the same thing so they, too, would be accepted. I've had men roll their eyes at me when I've suggested in a meeting we think about a different viewpoint. I've had them laugh in my face and dismiss me outright when I've suggested a course of action, only for two minutes later a man to suggest exactly the same idea and it suddenly be acted upon. I've had men call me after a meeting, asking me to explain my behaviour and suggest that I might consider being more "demure" and "serene" (two separate conversations from two different people. I remember these adjectives so distinctly). I've been asked to be less "passionate", too, apparently it was off-putting.

'Growing up, my mum (now 80) used to tell me about certain men. "They can't help it, it's just how men are. You just have to learn how to deal with it." And I did,' she goes on. 'I was brought up to believe that women always had to cover for men and not show them up. And I had absolutely bought into that and believed that's how you dealt with it. I continued this until around two years ago, when the #MeToo momentum was growing. It was like waking up from a coma and realising: *this is why it never stops*. Because we cover, we manage, we avoid, we circumnavigate, and we do not actively discourage men from being twats! And when we do, it is so abhorrent, so utterly shocking to them, that we are still the bad gals. Being called out rarely elicits a change of behaviour in men, it simply increases the rage that they feel towards women.'

The notion of just putting up with it really resonated for Juliet, 50, too. 'The making the tea (make it once and badly and they won't ask you again, someone once told me); the being told by a (female) mentor that I wasn't dressing correctly – I needed to wear a bright scarf to stand out at meetings; the time I spoke up at a board meeting and was told that I shouldn't have spoken out against my boss (even though what he was saying wasn't true) – and that perhaps I'd misunderstood the situation ...'

Alice, 51, has always taken a more robust approach to the men who dominate the management at her large corporation. 'I freely admit it's the result of being raised by a terrifying father and attending a very tough comp in south London where the boys shouted "Shut up, woman!" at us all the time. So nobody I ever worked with ever comes close, though they like to think they do.

'It makes me bridle. I have roared back at one very senior man, which, TBF to the ghastly old dinosaur, I think he respected. I have made a room full of men deeply uncomfortable again and again. Most of our high-level meetings are full of men called James, Andrew and Toby. I don't care what they think of me. I consider a high point of my career being told I was "abrasive" by a former boss ... He once told a colleague who was just back from maternity leave to "sit over there and look pretty".'

Paula has been on the trading floor at an investment bank since she was 22. 'I honestly loved it – the shouting, the banter, the stress, the pace, the adrenaline and the laughs,' she says. 'I was never bullied or sexually harassed – but I got married at 22 so it was always clear I had zero interest in any of them and I think I got a lot of respect for that. I am also very good at the sarcastic put-down, so most were too afraid to take me on. But when it came to my pay, it was nowhere even close – not even half what the men got. Even when I reached director level and I once raised an eyebrow at my bonus as I was disappointed (I'd had a cracking year), I was shouted at and told I should "count myself lucky, after all, what did nurses earn?" by my managing partner!'

Despite her level of seniority and success, Paula still admits to suffering from 'imposter syndrome and every day [I] expect a tap on my shoulder. I'm up for promotion and it's taken me years to get to a place where I know I can do it and I'm up against white men in their thirties ...'

Louise Nicolson, author of *The Entrepreneurial Myth*, tells a funny-not-funny story about telling her boss she was pregnant with her first son. 'I announced my news and he burst into a filthy grin and spontaneously, triumphantly, shouted: "You. Dirty. DOG!" He was as surprised as I was and quickly recovered himself, but it proved what lurked beneath. I've also had the usual humiliations of clients asking me to press the buttons on pitch presentations, assuming my male junior is somehow the lead. I've had clients asking me to staff their projects with the prettiest girls or lose their business (I refused and still kept their business). These things are like sedimentary rock – layer upon layer of indignities that both harden and strengthen me. This hard-won toughness separates us from younger women that thankfully, rightfully, work in different times.'

'It's only when we get to a more mature age that we are either able to stand up to these bullies – or have the stability financially to be able to walk away,' says Genevieve, who left her career in PR to start her own agency.

And many women do just that. Sick of playing the game, they start their own. But while that makes our own lives a fuck of a lot better, it doesn't do anything to change the wider working environment for women. On The Cut in 2015, journalist Lisa Miller wrote a passionate *cri de coeur* for more older women in the workplace. 'A good workplace is one in which you can look around and see versions of yourself five years from now, or ten. But for women, this exercise in mirroring gets harder and harder as they push towards 40, and 50, and beyond – for the simple reason that older women with ambition don't stick around. They dial back, drop out, start their own thing. They want more control, flexibility; they find themselves trapped in one more meeting, listening to one more self-serving anecdote by one more male superior who feels no urgency to head on home, and they reach their limit.'

Unfortunately, now, as then, the data on success and achievement in older women is appalling. Women over 40 are massively under-represented at the top of organisations. Take that to 50 and best not blink or you'll miss us. The pay gap between women and men in their fifties is 28 per cent and women can expect their salaries to drop by 8 per cent when they hit the big 5-0. When you add race to this picture the situation gets exponentially worse. Hardly any wonder we look for different ways to make work rewarding. Which is a shame because all the data shows that companies with at least one female senior executive are more likely to succeed than companies that have only men. Ditto venture-based start-ups with five or more women on board. In part it's about diversity – diverse businesses do better, period. But it's also back to the role model thing again. If young women can look up and see a future, how different might things be?

At the start of 2020, that future was looking tantalisingly close for some young women in the shape of candidate for the Democratic nomination for the US presidential election, Elizabeth Warren. In the space of just three primaries she went from serious contender to no-hoper. Her fall tells us a lot about how society still feels about women in positions of power. Despite her undoubted competence – or perhaps because of it – Warren was variously called 'sanctimonious', 'bossy', 'a narcissist', 'self-righteous', 'abrasive', 'intensely alienating' and 'a know-it-all'. Two women told FiveThirtyEight's Clare Malone that 'when I hear her talk, I want to slap her, even when I agree with her.' For real.

Her 'electability' was constantly held up to question. Why? Well, duh, sexism. But I don't think it's only sexism. I think it's ageism, too. Because the only thing worse than being a woman vying for a position of authority (and vying successfully if her annihilation of Mike Bloomberg in debate was anything to go by) is being an older woman vying for a position of authority. Warren was 70. She was also out of contention. Which left us with a battle for the Democratic candidacy between two white men who were both older than Warren: Bernie Sanders, 78, and Joe Biden, 77. (At the time of writing, Sanders has bowed out. So now the 2020 US presidential election will be, for the umpteenth time, between two affluent white male septuagenarians: Biden and Trump, 73.)

It's full-on misogyny. Speaking to Megan Garber for The Atlantic, Kate Manne, author of *Down Girl: The Logic of Misogyny,* says, 'Misogyny is the law-enforcement branch of patriarchy. It rewards those who uphold the existing order of things; it punishes those who fight against it.'

And one of the ways it punishes us is to call us bad names. To paint us as harridans, tyrants, controlling nags. Who hasn't been called bossy, difficult, stroppy, a pain in the arse, battleaxe, not a team player? Don't all fight to put your hands up. And don't get me started on infantilising phrases like GirlBoss. If anything was designed to make it clear that maybe girls *could* but women definitely *can't*, it was that ... The old rhyme may say that 'words can never hurt us' but they can do a helluva lot of the damage – financial, political, professional and moral – nonetheless.

Juliet has been called 'difficult', 'challenging', 'a bit scary'. Alice: 'abrasive'. Paula: 'I've been called gobby just because I answer back and am also bossy. No one would ever call a bloke bossy.'

'I'm not fucking bossy, I'm strong minded,' says Jenny. 'I'm not fucking difficult, I've got a different opinion to you, which I'm happy to dialogue, not claim as the right opinion. If you choose to see me as difficult or bossy, that, my friend, is *your* fucking problem.' She freely admits, though, that she wouldn't have been so free with her opinions even two years ago.

I was first called bossy boots long before I started school. Everywhere I looked – TV, film, children's books, in the playground, the classroom, everywhere – it was crystal clear that being bossy was A Bad Thing. Bossy little girls came to no good. It was only recently that I stopped being called those names – in fact, it was at almost exactly the point that I started to feel really comfortable with the fact of being them. So what if I'm bossy, opinionated, difficult, awkward? *So what?*

There's another thing women get called that broadly means the same thing: witch. Usually *old* witch. (See also crone and hag … Lisa Miller referred to herself as the resident crone, while Caryn Franklin is determined to reclaim 'cronehood'.) Because adding old to the negative doubles its offensiveness. Like bossy, aggressive, difficult, 'nasty' women, witches are women the patriarchy can't control. As Greer puts it in *The Change,* they are always: old, female; often: outlived husband or, worse, children; appear to have thrived at the expense of others (i.e. be old and not dead!). Calling someone a witch was a way of criminalising female power and discrediting female knowledge. Darcey Steinke makes this comparison in *Flash Count Diary*: 'The most common clues for demonologists though were connected to menopause. Chin hairs. Witch. Wrinkles. Witch. Warts. Witch. If a woman had on her arm a skin tag, then she was a witch. If in the presence of others a woman grew red and perspired heavily, then she was a witch. If in summer, unable to sleep, she wandered in her nightgown outside her house, then she was a witch. If she was quarrelsome, angry, spoke loudly and moved, at times, in quick bursts of chaotic energy to open a window or get a ladle of water, then she was definitely a witch.' Look at the way we now downplay our experience, just in case anyone notices the power we have stored up over the years and is too threatened by it. They – *we,* we might as well reclaim it

– are old, therefore we are unattractive and yet we have power that society doesn't understand ... To bastardise Tina Fey: like bossy women and bitches, witches get shit done.

One bossy woman/witch I've got a massive girl crush (witch crush?) on is the advertising legend Cindy Gallop. Gallop has made it her business to put herself and other women over 50 front and centre in both their public and private life. When she's not fighting ageism in advertising, she's running her start-up MakeLoveNotPorn. She's 60 now – a fact she posted all over her social media channels on her birthday – but she's long since been making it her business to broadcast her age. 'I tell everyone how old I am as often as possible. I consider myself a proudly visible member of the most invisible segment of our society: older women. I would like to help redefine what society thinks an older woman should look like, be like, work like, dress like and date like by the way I live my life,' she wrote in the *Guardian*. 'While ageism does exist in business, broadly speaking, older men are favoured over older women. Older men tend to be valued as "elder statesmen", whereas older women are seen as "past it", with simply no value.

'There is no substitute for experience. When you've been around the block a few times, you've encountered nightmare situations many times over. You know what to do when disaster strikes: you stay calmer, you handle it better – and you have an armoury of potential solutions at your disposal.

'Women get things done. We've always had to.'

Gallop's aim might be to 'reinvent what older women talk like, look like, fuck like', but the truth is we already talk and look and fuck like it. Society just doesn't reflect that. We are already growing louder, getting more confident and more secure. We just need society to acknowledge it. Or maybe what we just need is to give ourselves permission to not give a toss what society thinks.

'Everything I say about gender diversity is also true of race, ethnicity and sexuality,' Gallop goes on. 'Women challenge the status quo because we are never it.' She's right but that goes tenfold for women of colour, for instance, because for every insult, side swipe and undermining jibe I've tolerated, every black woman I know has tolerated dozens, if not hundreds, more.

Gallop is 60, loud and proud, and she's no longer alone. In just the time I've been writing this book I've seen more and more women of my age and older becoming increasingly vocal about how pissed off they are. (Inspired, I suspect, by the drive of younger women to have no more truck with putting up and shutting up.) And they're not about to put up with any more of that '50 is the new 30' BS. 'Sick of this 50 is the new ...' Minnie Driver, 50, tweeted earlier this year. '50 has always been 50. Women were previously expected just to shrivel and accept their husk. I suppose it must be terrifying to a lot of men if we actually burned brighter, hotter, more ambitious and emancipated from shame the older we got.'

Well, guess what? We already do. What's stopping us is our internal narrative. The one that's spent too many years listening to those voices that tell us we can't, we shouldn't, we aren't – and if we are it must be an accident. But things are changing, not just within us but externally, too. Better late than never, *Forbes* has just launched its first '50 over 50' list to highlight women 'shattering age and gender norms' (whose norms, I wonder ...). Sadly it's only open to women in the States. For now. And despite the woeful investment rates holding us back, women are starting more businesses than ever before with success rates improving as you get older. (I'm not saying start-up success is guaranteed; unfortunately I'm proof of that.) According to a study of 2.7 million start-ups (conducted by the US Census Bureau and two MIT professors), in general terms a 50-year-old entrepreneur is almost twice as likely to start an extremely successful company as a 30-year-old; a 60-year-old, three times.[41] Or, for that matter, a successful side hustle. We're back to seizing the means of production. 'Women have been taking control for centuries,' Kathy

McShane of the US Small Business Administration's Office of Women's Business Ownership, told *Inc.* 'But now we're talking about it.'

'At one time, fiftysomething meant the beginning of retirement,' wrote Candace Bushnell in *Is There Still Sex In The City?* 'Working less, slowing down, spending more time on hobbies and with your friends who, like you, were sliding into a more leisurely lifestyle. In short, retirement-age folk weren't expected to do much of anything except get older and a bit fatter and go to the doctor and the bathroom more. They weren't expected to exercise, start new businesses, move to a different state, have casual sex with strangers, get arrested, and start all over again, except with one-tenth of the resources and in many cases going back to the same social and economic situation that they spent all of their thirties and forties trying to crawl out of. But this is exactly what the lives of a lot of fifty- and sixtysomething women now look like.'

Geraldine, 57, is that woman. She went back to university last year, much to the confusion of her friends. 'I'm so fed up with the "at your age" thing,' she fumes. 'The majority of my friends have been incredibly supportive but a few have said, "but what can you do with a degree now?" My answer? "Whatever I fucking want!"' She goes on: 'Another thing I've had a lot of is, "So that's you retired then?" No it fucking isn't. I study 35 hours a week, I read on average another five on top of that, I volunteer 15 hours a week and am about to start a job five hours a week. Retirement? I think not.'

Geraldine, like Cindy, like me (I'm proud to say, although I can't pretend it's been easy or, indeed, fun), like countless others who decided they didn't like the rules of other people's games, have started to make their own. This is not a call to 'start that business from your kitchen table', unless that's something you've always hankered to do. Ditto if you've always wanted to take a pottery class, learn to code, write that book (or even a blog), build a website or start an Instagram that's about more than your cat. Volunteer if you've always wanted to, channel your inner activist, go back to school or sign up for a course. Invest in yourself.

In short, if you're sick to the back teeth of playing the game, go ahead and devise a new one, one where you make at least some of the rules.

'I'm no longer accepting the things I cannot change. I'm changing the things I cannot accept.'

Angela Davis

15

NEVER PICK A FIGHT WITH A WOMAN OVER 40. THEY ARE FULL OF RAGE AND SICK OF EVERYONE'S SHIT

You're going to get angry. Really really angry. Here's how to harness it

It was anger that got me here. (For good, or ill.) I see that now. Uncontained, untrammelled anger that caused something inside to snap.

I was 45 and arguably 'at the top of my game'. I'd been editing *Red* for a long time, sales were at their peak and I was desperate for a new challenge. I had been angling, cajoling and generally being the bane of my bosses' lives for several months, when an opportunity came up – *the* opportunity, in fact. The one magazine in the company I'd been desperate to get my mitts on for years. And so I started to jump through hoops. Tell me how high and I guarantee you I jumped higher. I applied formally. And I started spending every spare minute working on my vision for this other magazine. I knew plenty of other editors were also applying for it – the rumour mill was working overtime – but my track record was one of the best in the industry. I'd won awards, I'd boosted the sales and the ad revenues of almost every magazine I ever worked on (with one doomed exception) and already made millions and millions and millions for the company I worked for. I didn't think they owed me, because I wasn't brought up to believe anyone owes you anything, but I did think I stood a good chance. I discussed my ideas with my boss. He loved them. I emailed him through several documents full of ideas, at his request. He asked for more. I sent those, too. I did a formal interview, all mood boards and visions and brand extensions. I knew my ideas were good. I'm an introvert not an idiot and by then I had cured myself, largely, of raging imposter syndrome. This was my world. In this world I was not an imposter, of that I was sure.

Then he asked me to pop round to his office. I practically sprinted. I confess I thought I'd nailed it. Hubris is a terrible thing.

I'd like to transcribe the full conversation here for your reading pleasure, but TBH I can't remember it all. It's a red haze. But I remember one phrase: *'You do not come from the right background to edit a magazine like [insert your guess at the name of the magazine here].'* It's no exaggeration to say I felt the insult physically, like being punched in the gut. My vision blurred and, clichéd as it sounds, the room really did spin. I can't tell you what else he said because in my mind his voice took on the quality of the teacher in Charlie Brown. Wah-wah-wah. Less than five minutes later I was walking back along the corridor to my office, a different woman to the one who'd walked the other way, a bounce in her step, with no idea how I was going to get through the rest of the day. I didn't 'come from the right background'. What the hell did that mean?

He probably thought it had gone surprisingly well. (If he thought about it at all, which I doubt.) He probably congratulated himself and lined his multi-coloured Muji pens up by colour and nib size to celebrate, then asked one of his three PAs to make him one of his special coffees in one of his special cups. He'd dealt me a body blow and there'd been zero repercussions. I didn't talk back, I didn't argue, I didn't yell, I didn't storm out, I didn't demand he justify the most offensive and prejudiced thing anyone had ever said to my face in 25 years of working in magazines (and I've heard plenty). I didn't even (praise be) well up. I smiled. I nodded. I probably even fucking thanked him for his time. I didn't ask for my ideas back. I just left his office as soon as I could and plastered a smile on my face for the secretaries outside. I didn't even think 'fuck this shit' until at least five minutes later. Because that's what girls are raised to do. Smile sweetly, take it on the chin and carry the fuck on.

Except ultimately, this time, I didn't. I couldn't.

Within days I was sick, with a chest infection that quickly turned to bronchitis. I carried on working, because that was the kind of stupid thing I always did, going first to Milan and then to Paris for the fashion shows. I kept going. I even sat next to him at one of them. Bronchitis became chronic bronchitis, which ultimately became pneumonia. I finally stayed off work when the doctor signed me off for a week (I guess I needed someone else to give me permission to stay in bed, my own judgement, based on not being able to breathe, see or think, not being sufficient). Then I got MRSA – most likely from the three different types of increasingly strong antibiotics I was prescribed before the fourth managed to have some sort of impact. My GP phoned daily, but I wasn't admitted to hospital because 'it could prove fatal to people more vulnerable than you'. And by the time I fully returned to work, several weeks later, my body was in collapse. (My illness was somatic, of course – not that I recognised that at the time. My body had taken charge, physically displaying something my mind was unable to cope with.) That summer I had a deeply unpleasant operation that I'd been putting off for years that led to me spending a fortnight lying on the sofa watching the London Olympics off my face on Tramadol.

And when I recovered, I resigned.

I loved my job, I loved the magazine, I loved my team, I loved, if I'm totally honest, the status my job conferred on me. Although it was the kind of love you feel for something long-term and comfortable, but no longer exciting. But my fury wouldn't let me carry on. I'd gone over the top. I could not continue to leave my future in the hands of a man who looked at me and saw, not a talented professional with two decades' experience, but a working-class girl whose dad was a bricklayer and who'd gone to the local comprehensive. (Both things of which I have always been and always will be inordinately proud.) If I was not from the right background, my rage reasoned, then I was not from the right background to continue to make him millions of pounds on one of his most successful magazines. Let him find someone else to do it.

It's what the phrase 'the straw that broke the camel's back' was created for. It was created, I believe, for women who internalise and internalise and internalise. And then they snap.

I snapped.

There were other factors – of course there were. What was happening in the media for a start: it was 2012, the magazine industry was about to enter a period of unprecedented and irrev-ocable change and, at the time, very few people seemed prepared to face that; the fact I had a tentative idea for something new and different; the explosion of mobile; the fact that at my great age I felt I had one chance left to do something really different and meaningful.

I lost count of the number of people who told me how brave I was. How they would love to do the same. (Sensibly, they didn't. Although many of them went on to lose their jobs anyway, such has been the media landscape of the past decade.) But the truth is, I was in my mid-forties, the main earner in our family and I'd just made a unilateral decision to chuck in my job and, more urgently, my salary and go it alone without discussing it with everyone else who'd be affected by my decision to put a bomb under our life. (Something that has had fairly disastrous financial repercussions we are still dealing with eight years later.) But I couldn't not do it. Something bigger than me was driving me – and it drove me straight off a cliff. Years and years and years of pent-up rage. It was also, I suspect now, perimenopausal fury. I wonder how many other women in their forties and fifties feel the same right now.

Western culture in particular isn't comfortable with angry women. Anger is unseemly, it's not ladylike, it's not sexy. It's not fun. Angry men are just men, doing their big man thing and asserting themselves. Angry men are powerful. Angry women are a problem. But if there's one thing menopause gifts you it's a righteous fury, an indignation, an inability to suffer fools and unfairness and injustice that I used to write off as just 'how it was'.

Which brings me to anger, and the way women deal with it. (Or don't deal with it. Or are not allowed to deal with it.) And, more pertinently, the way our approach to it changes once we've gone 15 rounds with menopause. Before, if I was angry, I literally swallowed it down and occasionally it would overflow in meetings in the form of hot angry tears that made me look and feel pathetic. I turned my anger inwards, rather than direct my fury at its real target. I was, I guess, complicit. During perimenopause, though, my anger became erratic and, occasionally, terrifying. Now it's no less ample, but it's considered. And it's fierce, deeply felt and passionate. I rage at injustices in a way I haven't since I was an angry five-year-old. Or maybe younger. I'm inclined to think I'd already learnt to be A Good Girl by the time I was five.

I believe what a lot of perimenopausal rage is about is having spent 20, 25, 30, 40, even more, years keeping a lid on it, turning that rage inwards instead of railing outwards at the injustices around us. It's about being taught to be a good girl and staying that way – no matter how much the fury (or worse, resentment) builds inside, mutating into depression. Until, one day, maybe because our good friend oestrogen (the biddability hormone) wanes, or maybe just because one person can only take so much, we are aflame with righteous, uncontrollable, furious anger. It comes in bursts, it comes in waves, it comes in like a tornado, a tsunami, a volcano. We are incandescent. And it is out of our control. Suddenly, we are angry about everything.

WE ARE ANGRY ABOUT ALL THE CARING WE ARE ANGRY ABOUT ALL THE RESPONSIBILITY FOR BIRTH CONTROL WE ARE ANGRY THAT THE WORDS MOTHER AND WOMAN ARE OFTEN TAKEN TO BE ONE AND THE SAME THING WE ARE ANGRY ABOUT THE PAIN EVERY BLOODY MONTH WE ARE ANGRY ABOUT DOING ALL THE CHILDCARE AND HOUSEWORK AND PARENT CARE AND DOMESTIC LOAD-CARRYING WE ARE ANGRY ABOUT TAKING ALL THE CAREER RISK WE ARE ANGRY ABOUT BEING PAID LESS AND DOING MORE WE ARE ANGRY ABOUT BEING EXPECTED TO BE SEXY AND MATERNAL AND FECUND AND YOUTHFUL AND THIN BUT NOT TOO THIN AND CURVY BUT NOT TOO CURVY AND BASICALLY JUST VISUALLY APPEALING SO MEN GIVE US AIR TIME WE ARE ANGRY ABOUT ALL THE TIMES WE WERE TALKED OVER OR PUT DOWN OR UNDERMINED WE ARE ANGRY ABOUT BEING JUDGED AND FOUND WANTING WE ARE ANGRY ABOUT BEING MADE TO FEEL GUILTY ABOUT EVERYTHING ALL THE TIME WE ARE ANGRY ABOUT HAVING TO PROVE OURSELVES OVER AND OVER AGAIN WE ARE ANGRY ABOUT ALL THE THINGS WE'VE PUT UP WITH THAT WE KNOW WE SHOULDN'T HAVE PUT UP WITH BUT WE THOUGHT WE HAD TO WE ARE ANGRY ABOUT HAVING TO PRETEND ALL THE FUCKING TIME THAT WE'RE NOT ANGRY AND WE ARE ANGRY ABOUT HAVING TO SMILE SMILE SMILE LOVE IT MIGHT NEVER HAPPEN.

It's exhausting.

In *Rage Becomes Her*, award-winning journalist Soraya Chemaly asks, 'How many times does a woman say "I'm so tired" because she cannot say "I'm so angry"?' Chemaly is right that tired is a shorthand for angry, but many of us *are* tired, too. We are tired *and* angry, from all that putting up and shutting up and holding it in. Exhaustion plus anger equals resentment. And I wouldn't be surprised if it isn't eating us alive.

'Anger is a forward-looking emotion, rooted in the idea that there should be change,' says Chemaly. 'Resentment, on the other hand, is locked in the past and usually generates no meaningful difference in the situation.' We have all known people like this, usually older women in our lives, often women who've spent years living half-lives that have left them eternally disappointed. Women like my maternal grandmother, who by the time she was in her fifties and sixties her every pore oozed discontent. She was emotionally walled-up. With the benefit of hindsight, it's not that hard to see why. 'Resentment is like drinking poison and waiting for the other person to die,' quipped Carrie Fisher. And you know who does that? Women. If bitterness and resentment kill anyone, it's the person whose body is marinating in it. All those years of resentment are blown sky-high during perimenopause. Well, that's my theory. Certainly my years of resentment were. And afterwards? Afterwards you're left with healthy, productive, conscious anger. And take it from me, that's a good place to be. But first you gotta get there.

Angry women are dangerous women – or so society seems to think – so from an early age we're trained not to be. If we're angry, people won't like us, we're told. Even small children report finding anger in boys OK, whereas anger in girls is not, according to a review of anger and gender studies by Ann M. Kring, a psychology professor at Berkeley, in 2000.[42] In the same review, women's anger is more often described as bitchy and hostile, while men's is strong and powerful. Female anger is destructive, unnatural, a bad and unattractive thing. And so girls are trained to be nice. And good. To put up and shut up.

My family was no different. We don't do anger. We do disappointment. We do displeasure. We do sadness. We do atmospheres – as I've said earlier, my nan was an expert in icing the room if things weren't going the way she wanted. Since I was small I've been an expert in taking the temperature of a room almost before I walk in it. I still am, although I'm slowly (v-e-r-y slowly) learning that someone else's displeasure is not my problem to solve. Nan's mode of anger was cold, white-lipped fury. To this day I am terrified of that silent, tight-lipped anger. It throws me back in time to places I'd rather forget, setting me on high alert at the slightest change of facial expression. (Jon has often joked that he should have 'It's Just My Face' tattooed on his forehead.) Displeasure was exuded, not expressed; implied, inferred, emanated even – they don't call it passive aggression for nothing – and it is your responsibility – as the girl and the eldest – to identify the displeasure, discover the source and do your level best to make it go away. So I used to be able to say, with a twisted sort of pride, that we did not do anger in our family. I was taught to fear, ignore and hide it. We were not those kind of people. We were not angry by nature. We did not do seeing red. We did not – and still don't – do throwing or shouting or slamming or putting fists through walls. I don't think I ever heard my parents shout at each other – hiss, maybe. I never had the experience of Caroline, 55, who, as a younger woman, was a self-confessed people-pleaser and peace-keeper, 'probably due to having a very angry mother and growing up as an only child amidst frequent rows between my parents – screaming at night, crockery being thrown, rages and tantrums. All triggered by Mum. Dad was far from perfect (I think he might be on the spectrum), but he wasn't – and isn't – a shouter or instigator of rows. I once threw myself downstairs (probably aged about seven) to stop them rowing.'

Consequently, Caroline says, 'conflict horrifies me and I go to great lengths to avoid it.' But what really interested me about that was that I could put my hand on my heart and say, me too. I too have always been a people-pleaser and a peace-keeper, horrified by conflict and inclined to go to great lengths to avoid even the slightest confrontation (which does not make for a great management style, I have to admit). Though Caroline and I had totally different childhood experiences of expressions of anger, our outtake was the same: it was our responsibility, as girls, to make it better.

Stella, 48, experienced this in the extreme. 'At 13 years old, I picked my mother off the floor after an unsuccessful overdose attempt. She was sprawled on the lino, drunk from cooking sherry, holding a note I wasn't allowed to read. I was incandescent with rage that she had wanted to leave us. I was told: don't tell your sister, don't tell your grandparents, don't tell your teacher, don't tell your friends. *Don't, don't, don't.* But I did. I howled with raw fury. I ran away. I came back. I punished them all. I skipped school to drink peach wine in the park. I stole my stepmother's ID to dance in nightclubs. I sat at the front of class and laid my head on the desk and slept in full view of my beloved English teacher, daring her to wake me. I burned with a white-hot anger that curdled everything I touched. And the real tragedy is, my anger was made the problem. It was pathologised.'

It was the same teacher Stella had goaded – not parents or family or friends – who 'saved' her. 'She fixed her eye on me and told me I could write,' Stella says. 'She introduced me to Antoinette Cosway in Jean Rhys's *Wide Sargasso Sea*. She taught me there was always a backstory to the fury and madness and unfairness. And it doesn't always have to end up in the attic. If a girl or woman is angry, the emotion itself becomes the focus, the point, the problem. An end in itself. It's the freak show. Good girls swallow it. Never mind what sparked it.'

People recoil from angry women. Take Medusa, that classic angry woman whose backstory gives her and us plenty to be furious about. A human woman who was raped by Poseidon, she was turned into a gorgon as further punishment by Athena before being beheaded by Perseus. I mean, seriously, who wouldn't be livid?

According to Chemaly, 'Studies show differences between men's and women's experiences of feeling angry are virtually non-existent. [If anything] women report feeling more anger and for longer periods of time. Men associate anger with feeling powerful, while women associate anger with powerlessness.' And so, we learn to put aside anger to de-escalate conflict, to keep the peace, to avert violence, to minimise risk, and as girls and young women we are constantly making these assessments. This sounds like my life. Like many other women, it took me a long time – until now, in fact – to learn that everything is not my responsibility. Other people's feelings and behaviour are not all about me.

'A combination of growing up mixed race and female with (no judgement) an emotionally unwell single mother meant that it never felt safe to be angry, and so I just … wasn't. Outwardly,' says Karen, 50. 'Most of my esteem and survival came from reacting as softly as possible. As a younger woman, I only really allowed emotions when I drank and I, too, was an angry crier. I guess I genuinely was sad for many reasons unprocessed and logically filled with unexpressed rage.' Karen got sober at 31 but has only really learnt to express anger appropriately recently. 'I think I still got some of my self-esteem/feeling of superior control from "not being angry",' she admits.

We start undermining girls' right to feel 'unladylike' feelings at an early age. We tell them it's not cute, not nice, not ladylike to be angry, to be bossy, to be attention-seeking, to show emotion, and as they get older, to be ambitious, to seek power. When I was growing up, temper tantrums were not a thing to be tolerated, they were a thing to be punished. And so you kept your rage to yourself. But, even now, our toleration of angry little girls is limited once it stops being entertaining enough to put on Instagram or YouTube. By the time you're a teenager, being an angry girl is so not cute; it's simply not acceptable. And by the time you're a woman – unless you're a mother, in which case it's permissible to 'defend your cubs' – it's totally unattractive.

'Women are expected to express displeasure in sadness ... Whereas men express displeasure in anger,' says Chermaly. 'A sad woman and an angry man may be experiencing the same emotions. But anger is linked to assertiveness and aggressiveness and leads to perceptions of status and respect. Sadness doesn't.' Anger is powerful, sadness is powerless under greater scrutiny than those by men'. And so we go on. Maybe this is why so many of us cry in frustration when we're angry, when really we want to punch a wall? Try as we might, we just can't let the anger out, but sadness is OK, so we run to the loo and have a quick blub, furious with ourselves, before slinking back into the meeting, cheeks hot with shame and embarrassment.

Women who don't 'keep a lid on it' soon discover the repercussions of being an angry woman. We are 'crazy white women' or 'angry black women', we are 'nasty women' (to coin a phrase), we are hysterical (the madness label is never far from an angry woman), harridans, old bags, humourless feminists, we are deemed to have 'resting bitch face' (such a widely recognised 'medical condition' that you can even get a specific cosmetic surgery for it ...). Women who are direct and decisive in professional situations are likely to be considered cold, bitchy and hard, and unpopular with their employees, whereas men in the same situation are deemed strong and decisive. 'Both men and women are held to norms of appropriate emotional expression in the workplace, but emotional expressions by women tend to come under greater scrutiny than those by men,' write the authors of *Constrained by Emotion: Women, Leadership, and Expressing Emotion in the Workplace*, Jacqueline Smith, Victoria Brescoll and Erin Thomas. 'Women incur social and economic penalties for expressing stereotypical "masculine" emotions because they threaten society's patriarchal barriers against the "dominance of women"', they say. At the same time, when women behave in a more 'socially approved' way 'they are judged as lacking emotional control, which ultimately undermines women's competence and professional legitimacy.'[43] For men, anger is power-enhancing, for women not so much.

We're back to the old difficult-women schtick again. 'I have always understood that being seen as an "angry woman" – sometimes simply for sharing my thoughts out loud – would cast me as over emotional, irrational, passionate, maybe hysterical and a certainly "not objective" and fuzzy thinker,' admits Chemaly. 'I am constantly being reminded that it's "better" if women didn't "seem so angry". What does "better" mean exactly?'[44]

And better for who? Not us, that's for sure.

Is it any wonder so many women are passive aggressive? It's like that old joke, 'Mum won't be angry, she'll just be very, very disappointed.' We all grin and nod and laugh because we all know how it feels to have a scarily disappointed mum. But the reality is maybe Mum will be disappointed because she's never felt able to be angry? Maybe she's had to suppress her anger so it oozes out in the form of disapproval. Is it any surprise that so many women's anger manifests as stress and depression? That teenage girls nurture eating disorders, starve and cut themselves and act out? When you keep your anger inside you get ill, like I did.

According to Chemaly, 'Depression has been described as a "silent temper tantrum".' Globally women experience depression at seven times the rate that men do. Which brings me to shame. 'Women feel shame more than men, who are more inclined to say they feel guilt,' according to Chemaly's research. 'Guilt is the response of a person who feels he had some control and failed to exercise it properly. Shame reflects no expectation of control. It is a feeling that you, your essence and being are wrong.'

Which is why age-shaming is primarily a problem for women in perimenopause. 'As women approach and go through menopause, naturally gaining weight as fat-to-muscle ratios shift, they exhibit many of the same anxieties and symptoms that teenage girls do. The process of growing older makes women's [so-called] "flaws" more visible and acute; thus ageing, a natural process, becomes frightening, disorienting and difficult for many women. Suppressing anger and internalising objectification are as linked to middle-aged drops in self-esteem and increased mental distress as they are in younger girls and women.

'The anger and aggression women feel however can always be abated by an infinite list of beauty products, some of which have the added benefit of eliminating the appearance of anger entirely,' she goes on. 'Even if a woman is angry, no one should know it by looking at her face.'

Just at the point we are accumulating the power to push back, here comes the Botox! Seriously, though, you Botox if you want to. The point is more this: the more we internalise our anger, as we have been learning to do since we were knee high to nothing, the more it's going to blow when it finally comes out. Hence the peri-maelstrom.

Apart from that one time in that hotel room, I don't know if I had ever truly expressed anger before perimenopause – and the results were dramatic and had long-term consequences to say the least. That doesn't mean I wouldn't have made the same decision had I had more experience of feeling and expressing my own anger. But I certainly would have gone about it in a different way. When you've spent a lifetime subconsciously numbing yourself to your feelings, it's no surprise you're not sure what to do with them when they suddenly burst forth. 'My anger felt off the scale and uncontrollable when I was around 50 and peri. I used to drive alone, in the country, screaming with rage,' says Caroline. 'Perimenopause has absolutely floored me, anger-wise,' says Paula, 49. 'I have always been a little tornado when something really calls for it, but it's the inner swelling of rage that took me by surprise.' Deborah agrees: 'At around 43 I began to get big mood swings that turned into rages. Throwing things, screaming, like an out-of-body experience. It scared me, because I couldn't control them.'

Menopause is adolescence all over again, only you are an adult and have to go out into the world every day. What I think happens during perimenopause is that the lid finally comes off, or the cork pops, or whatever analogy works for you. Yes, the waning of oestrogen makes us weirdly ragey, but maybe we're also just fed up and sick of everything – the injustices, the crap-putting-up-with, the pressure to be good, the making excuses for other people, for men – and finally letting out everything we've kept inside when we find out that, to add insult to injury, menopausal women are treated like shit and hardly anybody knows what the fuck is going on. Everyone is an expert, but nobody knows when it starts or when it will stop. We don't know how long it will last. We don't know what it stopping will look like. (And yes, I *am* sure it wouldn't be like this if men had it.) We are judged for how we handle it or how we don't – do HRT, don't HRT, try to stay young-looking, don't try to stay young-looking – and now every insult that's lobbed our way is prefaced with 'old' or suffixed with 'for your age'. Is it any wonder we're angry?

As Jenny says, 'The rage is real. It's very hard to distinguish whether that's menopause or just the absolute shit state of the world at the moment. I suspect a little of both.'

There's a novel Germaine Greer cites in *The Change*, called *The Dangerous Age* – which is what menopause was also known as at the end of the 19th century. It's by Danish novelist Karin Michaelis and was translated into English in 1912. It wasn't easy to get a copy but I tracked one down and, to be brutally frank, the most interesting thing about it is the title. I don't have a problem with menopause being called the dangerous age; in fact I like it because the question that most interests me is who is it danger-ous for? Eleanor Roosevelt didn't say 'Anger is one letter short of Danger' for nothing. (If she said it at all. I do wonder if she really said everything that's credited to her ...) Because when we learn to use our anger, we become dangerous in the best possible way. 'The older I get, the more I see how women are described as having gone mad, when what they've actually become is know-ledgable and powerful and fucking furious,' wrote journalist Sophie Heawood in the *Guardian*. And she's right. An angry mid-life woman can be lethal.

In the wake of #MeToo, *The New York Times* ran a piece by Ruth La Ferla dedicated to older women's anger, entitled *They're Mad as Hell*. Anger, among older women (by which they meant 70+) was 'trending', they said. They were right, to a certain extent. Those women had probably been angry for a very long time. But #MeToo lit the fuse that told them it was OK. It was OK to be fucking livid at the things they had put up with their entire lives. 'At a certain age – psychologically, biogenetically, I don't know – you get to the place when a switch flips,' said Toni Tunney, who is in her seventies. 'You tell yourself, I'm done.' Paula Liscio, 71, agreed: 'Looking back on those years, I think, "Oh, we swallowed such a pile of garbage."'

I'm 20 years their junior, but didn't we just? Oh, the garbage we swallowed.

'I would say my anger as a younger woman was borne out of frustration and my anger now is borne out of incredulity and outrage,' says Jenny. 'As a younger woman I was regularly frus-trated by being talked over, not listened to, bypassed, laughed at – God, the laughing,' she shudders. 'And these responses trig-gered imposter syndrome. What if they were right and what I was saying *wasn't* credible, or correct, or valuable? And while I can remember angrily trying to push those thoughts down, the seed was definitely sown ... maybe there is some truth in what they're seeing in me. Back then, my anger would come out by crying bitterly on the way home at a) my ineptitude at dealing with the situation in the moment and b) the fact I'd probably exacerbated the perception of me not quite being up to the mark.'

How familiar is that? I was dogged by a constant sense of shame and blame through my teens and into adulthood. That my opinion wasn't valid, that things were 'all in my imagination', that I was, in fact, not worthy of a place at the table. It's not a million miles from the old angry woman as mad over-sensitive hysteric trope that has gaslit women for centuries.

'My anger has been received with clichés by men that it's an overreaction, that my experience isn't what it is,' says Karen. 'But I think it took me so long to allow myself to express anger that the advantage now is I trust my own screening process. If I'm angry it's probably with credence.'

Stella, 48, has tried to take a lesson from the anger-confident men around her. 'For men, anger is fuel, drive, passion,' she says. 'It's the means. It's the cheering audience. My husband has taught me about anger. He's not afraid of it as it rolls up and over and away. There is no aftertaste, no shame; just noise. It has driven him to move and build and change. It's a lifelong lesson to allow anger to do its work. That's why I think it's easier as we age. I am less inclined to numb anger with wine, to run away from it or weaponise it to hurt others. I look sideways at my husband and try to hold the line as he does.'

Many of the women I spoke to said they felt their anger now – late forties and beyond, but very much depending on where they were in their own menopause – was part and parcel of who they are. An acceptable emotion that they harnessed in just the same way as they would harness any other emotion. Not an emotion that controlled them. But one that they controlled and used for what they considered worthwhile ends.

'I still rage against the things that I consider unjust ...' said @Misssnowdome on Instagram. 'But the outbursts that came with menopause have lessened. Six years post-menopause I do feel calmer in myself ... I pause and breathe. I'm learning the art of letting it pass.'

'What used to make me angry and tied me up in knots, was stuff that I can now speak up about and be proactive in dealing with,' added @dollydonegal. 'Finally a benefit of menopause!'

'What's changed lately is that I have been able to stand behind the stuff that warrants my anger and express it regardless of the "angry black woman" trope,' Karen told me. 'I choose my battles but once I have, I don't need sign-off as to their validity. Now I'm kind of all war or none of the war! I'm angry about racism, sexism, how we treat and view the vulnerable, dishonesty, inequality. I always was, but before I couldn't express it ... I'm no longer angry about petty whispers in my industry, being in or out, who's got what, etc. But I am angry that women still have to prove themselves more than once, that I am constantly covering for men I report to whose roles are secure. I'm angry that my skin colour adds a negative bonus point to this situation *and* being told that it doesn't '

'I am still an angry woman,' says Stella, not without a hint of pride. 'Quick to flare up, noisy, often outraged – but I like this bit of me. It's protected me and propelled me on. I have been seriously ill and I think over the past 18 months, it's not an outrageous exaggeration to say it's helped keep me alive.'

For me and many of the women I spoke to this new post-menopausal anger is like rocket fuel. It keeps us going and powers us on, but we are able to turn it on and off, if not at will then almost. And, most importantly, we are able to move on. Not fret and ruminate and cogitate on what we said or did or shouldn't have done. It boils down, I think, to experience. (That much under-rated quality.) Driven by years and years of evidence that we are not imagining it, making it up or making a fuss about nothing, experience tells us to pick our battles and, once chosen, fight those battles hard.

Despite saying she's far more tolerant than she has ever been, Alice refers to having a new-found 'menopausal superpower' at work. 'A colleague took to Twitter to slag me off yesterday,' she told me. 'Not by name, but still. He has been forced to apologise but I am really looking forward to making him do it in person and making sure he knows just how much this confirms my already low opinion of him. I'll do it face-to-face, not in public, but then I am a grown-up. As soon as it happened I called my big bosses who, to be fair, understood I wanted instant action. At another time in my life I might have felt wounded, but this time I was glowing with rage. And I used it. This is an excellent example of our menopausal superpower.'

That 'menopausal superpower' can be used to make our own lives better and those of others – something that has never been more important as the world ebbs and flows around us in completely unforeseeable ways. 'I want to use this energy to effect change,' says Jenny. 'To create discourse and have better-quality conversations. This isn't just pointing and hissing about how shit it all is, it's asking, what do you think about this? If we did nothing about this, would that be OK in a year's time? Or five years' time?'

Grace Woodward agrees. 'I think anger is an incredible energy. One that I'm no longer ashamed of, one that I thought growing up was something that made me wrong or faulty. Now I realise how frightening it is because it's an expression of real female power. I have the energy and the will not to lie down and become a decoration that can silently be retired. What's great about anger is as I get older I know how to use it better. I'm no longer afraid of harnessing it as a positive not a negative.'

In *Flash Count Diary*, Steinke puts it like this: 'One of the clear gains of menopause has been a resurgence of my fierce little girl self ... my sense of injustice is sharper and I want to resist.'

For me, I was not such a fierce little girl – too well-behaved for that – so the rage I feel now is new but welcome. It makes me wonder what I could have done differently if I'd known what anger was and felt more comfortable using it when I was younger. But no matter. I know now and I have the life skills and the resilience to use it consciously and productively. And it's the conscious, productive use of anger that gives it its power. Power that, as women who grew up in the seventies, eighties and nineties, we might not be used to having.

It makes the future brighter than it might otherwise be – both for us and for the women coming after us. We are standing up for ourselves, we are putting ourselves if not first then nearer the front, we are speaking our minds. 'Angry woman' might have been an oxymoron to our mothers and their mothers and their mothers, too, but whether it's the hormones or whether it's the social change that has seen a generation of young women say 'we're not putting up with this shit' and made us wonder why the hell we had been, we are a new generation of angry women and we know how to use it. So let's channel that anger productively, let's work with young women, not against them. It's time to change.

'Fear, to a great extent, is born of a story we tell ourselves, and so I chose to tell myself a different story from the one women are told. I decided I was safe. I was strong. I was brave. Nothing could vanquish me.'

Cheryl Strayed

16

BRAVERY: A PERSONAL ESSAY

This is hard to write, but I'm going to write it.

Thirty-plus years ago, I was assaulted. (Not once, but repeat-edly.) By someone I loved or thought I did. By someone who was meant to love me. By someone whose cruel face and mean mouth I can still see when I close my eyes, and sometimes when I don't. By someone whose face I saw in the pursed lips and entitled fury of Brett Kavanaugh when he non-testified before the Senate committee. Someone whose voice echoed through my head when Kavanaugh answered every question with a question, alternating between mockery, insults, belligerence, whining self-pity and cold fury. And then, when that had barely subsided, vibrated through my skull again when the president of what we laughingly call the free world mocked Christine Blasey Ford in front of thousands of supporters the week after.

That was not how I originally planned to start this chapter. I had a whole other intro planned – something glib about balls and growing a pair, and why are all the bravery analogies so macho and linked to male genitalia, and that fabulous Betty White quote (if it was actually Betty White): 'Why do people say grow some balls? Balls are weak and sensitive. If you wanna be tough, grow a vagina. Those things can take a pounding.' But then, as I was lying awake at 3am worrying about all those things we worry about at 3am, my internal therapist – we'll call her Tessa, because that was, in fact, my therapist's name – woke up and gave me a good talking-to.

'Stop diverting,' she said. 'What did we say about shame?'

She was right. She is always right. How could I write about the courage menopause brings without writing about the worst thing that ever happened to me and the bravest thing I've ever done? That wouldn't be brave, that would be behaving the way I did for 30-odd years. That would be cowardly. Because as you now know, the worst thing that ever happened to me happened over 30 years ago now. And yet, it took me that long to find the courage to confront it. In autumn 2018, a year on from the opening of the floodgates that were #MeToo, a month after the lightning bolt that was the testimony of one of the bravest women I can think of, Dr Christine Blasey Ford, I wrote a piece for The Pool's subscribers. The beginning of that piece started this chapter. Here's a bit more:

For a year, almost to the day, we've all lived with #MeToo. For a year, we've talked about it daily, written about it almost as often, documenting each new case. And I've watched my friends and colleagues, seen signs of struggle, their spur-of-the-moment dashes from the room, and wondered how many of them are battling their own #MeToo.

In that year, watch is all I've done. I might have hashtagged #MeToo and #whyididntreport and #BelieveWomen. (Because, I didn't think anyone would believe me and because I thought it was my fault for having had sex with him in the first place, for staying when he hurt me and, worse, going back after I'd finally plucked up the courage to leave.) And I've cried in public toilets all over the country, but nothing like as much as I would have done if I'd not spent the last few years (finally!) having therapy to deal with PTSD, following a series of operations that dealt with the physical effects but left the mental ones unmended. That therapy dug the horrors out of the corners of my mind into which I'd bundled them. Rooms in my head reflecting endless other rooms ...

But I have not spoken out.

Then came the laughter, and all the horrors I thought had, if not gone away, then been reduced to something I'd become able to live with and largely ignore day to day, resurfaced.

The laughter. The mockery. The contempt. For her, for you, for me. The confirmation that even if they do believe us – if, big if – they don't really care. The confirmation, as if it were needed, that we don't really count ...

So, for now, I'm stopping here. This is as much as I can manage.

Thirty-plus years ago, I was assaulted by someone who was meant to love me. It has affected my life. My relationships. My marriage. I thought it was my fault. I know now it wasn't. I thought no one would believe me. Some people still won't. Right now, I can't face the inquisition. But I will. Because I remember. Like Ford, I don't remember every beer, every party, every drive, every date, every locked hotel room. But I remember. And, like all other survivors, I will never forget.

For more than 30 years, I hid. Or, more accurately, my mind hid from what it knew had happened to me in my teens. Truthfully, I (by which I mean my consciousness) didn't want to know the details. Oh, I knew I was fucked up. I suspected I dissociated – I had huge blank spots in my memory. Not days or weeks. It's not *Sybil*. (The Emmy-award-winning Sally Field film about a woman with multiple personalities, based on the book of the same name.) But certainly minutes and even, very occasionally, hours. I knew I had issues; like many women I struggled with food and body image and self-loathing, self-esteem, self-confidence and self-respect. When I didn't think I was the second coming, I thought I was a piece of shit. There was nothing in between. I knew I'd been raped and abused and undermined and coercively controlled in my teens and let down over and over again. Trust issues didn't even begin to cover it. 'You've made your bed, now lie in it,' was one of those things that was bandied around in the seventies. I took it literally now. I'd never found it easy to make friends. I always suspected I was not likeable, let alone loveable – but now I had proof; if I was, would this have happened to me? (Utterly illogical, I know.) Letting people anywhere near me emotionally became impossible. I was occasionally triggered (I say all this with the benefit of hindsight, of course). I freaked out to the point of becoming aggressive if anyone vanished into a blind spot behind me. To this day the sense that there's someone lurking behind me makes anxiety rise inside me, but at least I know it and no longer have to suppress the urge to lash out. I would occasionally find myself howling in the ladies with no idea why or how I got there. I had a pathological hatred of small rooms, particularly hotel rooms. Restaurants were problematic, too. I was hyper-alert to changes in mood and temperature and facial expressions. I picked away at non-existent scabs, causing rows to erupt that never would have happened if I hadn't 'foreseen' their coming and 'decided' I had no choice but to 'head them off' by starting them.

I didn't dream. I never dreamt. Sleep was a deep, dark pit – a respite I confess I loved and would vanish down at every available opportunity. It's a cliché to talk about sleep's welcoming arms, but that's how it felt. A blind, warm, cocooning escape from who knew what. The only negative waking up at the end of it. Oh, how I loved to sleep. I could turn off my consciousness at the drop of a hat. It was the ultimate refuge. Except for the nightmares. They were infrequent but horrific. I would wake screaming and gasping and suffocating and thrashing. More often I wouldn't wake. It would go on and on and on until Jon, becoming afraid for me, had to wake me, sometimes taking what felt like whole minutes to get me to surface, terrified, sweating, crying. And the night-mares were always the same. I was trapped in a small windowless room. I was terrified of whatever waited outside. Of whatever they had in store for me. If or when I ventured out, I was chased. I had the same nightmare for 30 years.

When you have been abused by someone who is meant to love you, you think – consciously or otherwise – you will never feel safe again. I lived life at arm's length, except for the occasional head-on collision. I will be eternally grateful that somewhere inside me I had the common sense to have one of those head-on collisions with Jon. A long dark night of the soul when we were very first together, when my sleepy brain dumped the whole ugly story on him as we lay in the dark. Six hours he said it took. Through the night into the dawn. When I woke the next morning I truly didn't remember telling him. (Sounds self-serving, doesn't it? But I swear it wasn't.) He, kind soul that he is, repeated the bare bones back to me, shouldering the rest alone. Until I faced up to the whole truth for myself, with the help of the legend that is Tessa, around the time I was 50.

It blows my mind just writing that sentence. I was 50. Thirty years turned inward. Thirty years closed down. Thirty years of being extremely difficult to live with. *Thirty.*

I write all that with the benefit of hindsight – and the best part of two years' treatment for PTSD. Before that I wouldn't have known a trigger if it slapped me in the face – which it often did. I didn't recognise almost any of these things when they were happening and I certainly didn't realise that I hadn't had an actual ordinary dream since my mid-teens. Until I had therapy, all I knew was shame. I thought what happened to me was my fault (I slept with him. I stayed with him. I even went back to him). I thought no one would believe me if I told them. I thought I was to blame. 'You were a teenager,' Tessa said, over and over again. 'You were a child. He was a grown man. You were not to blame.' It was the day I could look her in the eye and say I truly

273

believed it that I knew I was ready to go it alone again. But it was the day almost two years before that, when I asked my gynaecologist Claire, who had already helped me undo much of the physical damage of that 'relationship', to recommend a psychiatrist that I committed my first act of bravery as an adult.

But how did I get there? How did I finally find the courage to confront something that had had such a detrimental effect on my life and my relationships with other people? And what took me 30 years? I am as sure as it is humanly possible to be that the answer to the first two questions is perimenopause. Perimenopause and anger and that last operation. (I'll explain in a minute.) The answer to the third, of course, is trauma. And as all survivors know, you can't deal with trauma until you're ready to. No one else can make you. Until that point I would not have had therapy if my life had depended on it. (I can see now that it kind of did.) It had been suggested once or twice before and I had reacted with derision or anger or both. What did I need therapy for? Therapy was woo-woo and ding-ding and not for people as together as me. Ho ho. The point is, if someone doesn't see they have a problem, you can't make them see they have a problem. I say that as the person with the problem.

You already know what triggered it: the explosion of anger I wrote about at the start of the last chapter. That was the straw that broke the camel's back, but straws only break things when they're so over-burdened they're on the point of breaking anyway. I see now I had been teetering at that point for many, many years. Decades. (The breakdowns and the periods of somatic illness could be a bit of a clue.) And then I was ill and then I got better, sort of, and went back to work. Hating my boss, hating my job (poor job, it was not its fault, it was a wonderful job), hating myself. But more than that, something inside me had broken. My digestive system – for want of a better way of putting it – had packed up. Nothing worked. I was literally holding everything in; physically and emotionally clenched.

I had an operation. The last of a series to fix front, back and in between. And when I came round from the general anaesthetic I realised I was no longer in pain. Only I hadn't known I was in pain until I wasn't, because it turned out I had been in pain for the previous 30 years. It was my normal. My everyday. It lived at the heart of me.

The lifting of that physical pain was enormous; shocking. It changed me, it changed my life, it changed the lives of everyone around me. But to begin with I didn't know what to do with pain-free me, so for a long time I floundered. I experienced huge highs and catastrophic lows. Always a jay-walker, I lost count of the times I walked out in front of oncoming traffic. 'Accidentally.' My brain on other things, I told myself.

Then, not long after The Pool launched, a freelance writer filed the most incredible piece about being raped by a relative as a child. It was candid and brave and heartbreaking and remains one of the pieces I am most proud of on The Pool. And suddenly I was in the ladies in floods of tears, but for the first time in my life I came to crying in the loo and I knew why. Two weeks later I was huddled in an armchair in a psychiatrist's office, my entire body clenched onto the seat, closed in on myself, body language telling him everything he needed to know as I struggled through his questions. He prescribed antidepressants (which I had always, in the past, been too judgemental to take) and told me about a CBT therapist, Tessa Fane, who specialised in PTSD. At first I was dismissive (and terrified). PTSD was for people who were seriously traumatised – people who had seen war, terror and mutilation – not middle-aged women like me. (Wrong, of course. 10 per cent of women are likely to suffer PTSD in their lifetime as a result of rape, sexual assault or sexual abuse, 4 per cent of men as a result of physical assault, accidents, disaster, combat or seeing death or injury.[45]) He fixed me with a firm but not unfriendly gaze and told me he would contact her.

275

That was how I met Tessa. And, yes, the patient before me *had* just come back from Afghanistan and quite possibly the patient afterwards, too, but trauma takes on many forms and it took Tessa to make me see that what I had gone through – years of being hurt and hated at the same time as being told I was loved – was trauma. It was not just trauma, it was complex trauma because there was not just one incident to uncover and deal with, there were many, each one stored away deep in my brain out of sight, out of mind, or so I thought, but in reality each one able to jump out and cosh me whenever it fancied; each connected to the last. You read about the final one, way back in Chapter 2.

I saw Tessa weekly for the best part of two years and there were many times I left in floods, railing that I was never going back, that I didn't care if I never saw her consulting room ever again. But in the end, slowly, kindly, forgivingly, it was where I unpicked myself and faced up to things and ultimately put myself back together. I want to say Tessa did it but the truth is she didn't. I couldn't have done it without her but the person who rebuilt me was not her, but me. And thank God I did, because I don't know how I would have lived through #MeToo and the sexual assault allegations that came thick and fast if I hadn't.

I have never been particularly brave. Not until then, and not massively so since. I'm no Rose McGowan, although I live in awe of her and all the other women who spoke up and added their voice to hers in the battle to bring Harvey Weinstein to some sort of justice. But bravery doesn't have to be that bold. Bravery can be big or small – it can be standing up for what we believe is right, it can be not cowering from confrontation (as I have done too many times to mention), it can be having an argument you know needs to be had, it can be speaking up for people worse off than ourselves. It can be choosing to bite your tongue when you feel the moment is right. It can be making a decision and sticking with it. It can be saying no when you know no is the right thing to say, regardless of whether anybody listens. But still, we call other

people brave at the slightest thing. Some people truly are. Some
not so much. Most of us are occasionally and occasionally not. We
confuse small acts of kindness or of being true to ourselves with
big acts of courage. In the main, bravery is bigger, bolder, more
intentional; it's about looking the monster in the eye and saying,
OK, do your worst. And that was when I knew I was brave. I had
been brave before. Just once when I unlocked that bathroom
door and walked out, delivering myself into the hands of the
person who hurt me. For a long time, I feared that was cowardly,
it was stupid, it was giving up. But it wasn't. It was brave. It was
taking back control. It was saying do your worst, I won't put up
with this any more. And I believe I was brave, again, when I left
Red – even if I didn't do it in the most considerate way for those
around me. I took back control. I said I wouldn't – couldn't – put
up with it any more.

There were 30 years between those two incidents. It took me
30 years to find my way back to me. And now I've decided to be
brave again: I'm telling you about it. Because by telling you, I
might help you see how brave you can be, too.

'After a while, you've collected a bit of history. But rather than freaking out about it, I choose to honour it.'

Neneh Cherry

17

IT'S TIME TO WRITE OURSELVES A NEW STORY

And so here we are, out the other side – and somewhere along the line, when we weren't looking, when we were too busy worrying about the sweat or the flesh duvet or what the fuck age-appropriate meant anyway, and whether or not we cared, we shifted. The confusion and bewilderment, the anxiety and the hormonal haze, the what-the-fuck-is-the-point-of-me-ness that came along with perimenopause? Suddenly, it's gone – along with the blood and the killer cramps and ten quid plus every month on tampons – and what's left is the essence of us. With our confidence and our constructive anger and our disposable(ish) income and our knowledge that whatever life throws at us we can survive it, because ... we already have. And we've bounced back. And – you know what? – they can take their own notes and make their own bloody tea because, in all honesty, we can't be bothered. Call it wisdom, call it experience, whatever you call it, we've got it and it's a powerful force.

But we are missing one crucial thing: a narrative. We are, for the moment, storyless. Or, as I prefer, story-free. If, as far as society is concerned, women's usefulness really does end with happy ever after – house, husband, babies, all that – what next? After all, that story was written a long time ago and, even if you do choose to live your life that way, it only takes the first 40-odd years. So what about the next 40?

OK, so there are off-the-peg options you can try if you really fancy, but they're unlikely to fit the you who you've become today. It's called the old crone story; or its perkier sister the old lady who wore purple and rode a scooter; or cuddly accommodating granny who always has sweets in her pocket and nothing better to do than babysit. But come on, seriously, would you don one of those when you could be spirited, rebellious, fearless, vibrant? Or, if that sounds a bit too much like hard work (I hear you), how about just a stronger and more confident you, one that takes a lot less shit than you used to?

The only way we can change the boring, dismissive and predictable narrative of how older women are treated is to change it ourselves. Nobody else is going to do it for us. Why would they? There's nothing in it for them. So let's take those words that are wielded against us, the words that are used to subconsciously or otherwise write us off, and reclaim them: crone, witch, doyenne, grande dame, old bag, old bird (my personal favourite). What's wrong with them? Nothing. We only think so because we're told so. Just as we're told young is hot and old is not. Like anything, if you're told it often enough you start to believe it. As Kristin Scott Thomas said in a recent interview, 'Youth has its own beauty. So does age. It's just less fashionable, less celebrated. We don't celebrate maturity, we don't celebrate wisdom, there is an appetite for discovery and not much reflection on what you have accumulated along the way.' Who knew Kristin Scott Thomas would turn out to be The Shift's spirit animal?

There are countless stories to choose from, now you don't have to be the princess waiting to be saved. Be a witch, if you want to; claim your inner tribal elder, your oracle, your sage, or reclaim your former self, the little girl you used to be – the tree-climbing, game-playing, sweet-eating kid; or a new you, a combination of all three, outspoken, energetic, inquisitive, engaged, but with all the power and experience and resilience of your grown-up self. Or by all means, grab that smock and your dog and your knitting and make yourself comfy. Why not? There are as many stories to be written as there are women. We just need to give ourselves permission to choose the one that calls our name.

And then we should celebrate it, shout it from the rooftops, tell younger women there's no need to approach this time of life with the fear we did. 'If menopause happened to men there would be celebrations and parties every time one of them completed the change,' says Marian Keyes. She's right. There is no public rite of passage: no baby shower, no hen night, no divorce party, not even a wake! There's nothing else even half so momentous that you wouldn't throw a big old bash for. Big birthdays, anniversaries, even house moves and dogs' birthdays at least get acknowledged. Allow menopause to become a rite of passage and you make it something to celebrate, look forward to, even; an achievement, not a failing – a bridge to cross, not an abyss to fall down; a group to which suddenly women might aspire to belong instead of learning to dread.

And when we've finished celebrating this necessary rite of passage, let's grasp the shift in our lives to harness our energy for what really moves us. We may be 45, 50, 60 or beyond. We may no longer be able to reproduce (if we ever were) but this new us has a new power – a 'wise anger' as Soraya Chemaly calls it. And why wouldn't we? We have freedom, we have independence, we have experience, we have suffered and survived, we have resilience, we have the authenticity that comes with being 50 and really, truly not giving a fuck, except about the people and things we care about. The detritus is falling away, the people who drain us, who take take take. We have an invisibility cloak we can pull on and shuck off at whim, we can be visible to those who matter to us when we want to; the rest of the time, so what? Some of us may have a new-found sexuality, others may have embraced the power of can't be bothered. Our power might not be a power a patriarchal society recognises or values – it may not be the power of boardrooms and FTSE 100s – but it's potent and it scares them nonetheless. Because, you know, if you want something doing ... ask a mid-life woman.

Let's write ourselves a story we want to be part of. Let's have fun, be rebellious, cause trouble. Be whatever we want to be. We have power, we have freedom, we have half of our lives to live. And for the first time ever, nobody's checking up, nobody's monitoring, asking us when, why, how and what's for tea.

Nobody's watching. We're free!

EPILOGUE

Things I wish I'd known
(an homage to Nora Ephron)

Fifty is not the new thirty. It just isn't.

That back fat is not going anywhere, any time soon. Unless it's
your full-time job to make it do so.

You will always behave like a teenager when you're with your
parents.

That thing about white wine making you nauseous and giving you
the hangover from Hades? It's true. Still, there's always red.

Spanx is a 21st-century instrument of torture.

Nothing fits as good as happy feels.

You will never please your mother.

If you play them at their own game, you'll lose. It's *their* game.

A moisturiser is just a moisturiser. It moisturises. That's it.

There's more than one way to have sex.

It's OK to not have sex if you can't be arsed.

It's OK to not do anything if you can't be arsed. (Although possibly
not indefinitely.)

Think what you can do with the money you're not spending on
tampons.

If your heart says no, it's probably right.

Not all feelings are good. They're still allowed.

There's no such thing as a guilty pleasure.

You don't have to 'just put up with it'.

ENDNOTES

1 NHS (2019) 'Study Suggests HRT carries higher risk of breast cancer than thought'. Available at: www.nhs.uk/news/cancer/study-suggests-hrt-carries-higher-risk-breast-cancer-thought.
2 Germaine Greer, *The Change* (London: Bloomsbury, 2018) p.35.
3 Brigid Moss 'The Truth about Expensive Bioidentical HRT', *MPowered Women.* Available at: https://mpoweredwomen.net/medical/the-truth-about-expensive-bioidentical-hrt/; Julie Ryan Evans (2018) 'Bioidentical Hormone Replacement Therapy', Healthline. Available at: https://www.healthline.com/health/bioidentical-hormone-replacement-therapy.
4 Jeanette Winterson (2014) 'Can You Stop the Menopause', *Guardian.* Available at: www.theguardian.com/books/2014/apr/11/jeanette-winterson-can-you-stop-the-menopause.
5 Gillian Anderson and Jennifer Nadel (2017) 'The Truth is Out There (About Menopause)', *Lenny Letter.* Available at: www.lennyletter.com/story/the-truth-is-out-there-about-menopause.
6 Transparency Market Research (2016) 'Menopausal Hot Flashes Market to Reach US$5.28 bn by 2023, Estrogen Leads Hormonal Products in Revenue and Prescription Volume', *Cision PR Newswire.* Available at: https://www.prnewswire.com/news-releases/menopausal-hot-flashes-market-to-reach-us528-bn-by-2023-estrogen-leads-hormonal-products-in-revenue-and-prescription-volume-564235661.html.
7 Maya Oppenheim (2019) 'Menopausal women often prescribed antidepressants which make their symptoms worse, warn experts', *Independent.* Available at: www.independent.co.uk/news/health/menopause-antidepressants-symptoms-worse-hrt-shortage-a9148951.html.
8 Emma Hartley (2019) 'How to Delay the Menopause: can this

surgery postpone "the change", *Sunday Times*. Available at: www.thetimes.co.uk/article/ how-to-delay-the-menopause-can-this-surgery-postpone-the- change-xqt79tc3w.

9 Suzanne Moore (2015) 'There Won't Be Blood', *New Statesman*. Available at: www.newstatesman.com/lifestyle/2015/08/there -wont-be-blood-suzanne-moore-menopause.

10 ANAD (2020) 'Eating Disorder Statistics'. Available at: https:// anad.org/education-and-awareness/about-eating-disorders/ eating-disorders-statistics.

11 NHS (2017) 'Eating disorders in middle-aged women "common"'. Available at: www.nhs.uk/news/mental-health/eating-disorders -in-middle-aged-women-common.

12 Anne Pietrangelo (2018) 'Eating disorders plaguing older women', Healthline. Available at: www.healthline.com/health- news/eating-disorders-plaguing-older-women.

13 Dominic-Madori Davis (2020) `Ignoring older consumers in favor of courting millennials and Gen Zers could cost the fashion industry over $14 billion in the next 20 years, new research says', *Business Insider*.

14 Darcey Steinke (2019) 'No One Told Me Exactly What to Expect From Menopause. But the Messages I Did Get Were Very Wrong', *Time*. Available at: https://time.com/5616247/menopause- expect-messages/.

15 Bruce Handy (2016) 'An Oral History of Amy Schumer's "Last Fuckable Day" Sketch', *Vanity Fair*. Available at: https://www. vanityfair.com/hollywood/2016/05/amy-schumer-last-fuckable-day.

16 Kieron Connolly, *Dark History of Hollywood*. (London: Amber Books, 2017)

17 Monica Corcoran Harel (2020) 'Hollywood's Menopause Problem: "The Silence Around It Perpetuates Silence Among Women"', *Hollywood Reporter*. Available at: www.hollywood- reporter.com/news/women-hollywood-talk-menopause -1271507.

18 Hannah Devlin (2020) 'Having more sex makes early menopause less likely', *Guardian*. Full article available at: www.theguardian. com/science/2020/jan/15/having-more-sex-makes-early-meno- pause-less-likely-research-finds. Findings are based on 2,936 women aged on average 45 recruited into a US menopause study

called the SWAN cohort in the 1990s. None of the women had entered menopause, but 46 per cent were starting to. By the 10 -year follow-up, 45 per cent had experienced a natural meno- pause at average age 52.

19 *The Change* p.63.
20 *The Change* p.100.
21 *The Change* p.114.
22 Hamoda H, Panay N, Arya R, Savvas M (2016) `The British Menopause Society & Women's Health Concern 2016 recommen- dations on hormone replacement therapy in menopausal women', *Post Reprod Heal* 22(4):165 -183.Survey by Rest Less for ONS, reported in the *Guardian*: Amelia Hill (2019) 'Gender pay gap at its widest for women in their 50s'. Available at: https://www. theguardian.com/world/2019/oct/28/gender-pay-gap-at-its- widest-for-women-in-their-50s-study-reveals.
23 Imali Hettiarachchi (2018) `Dear White Men, We Need You', *Campaign*. Available at: www.campaignlive.co.uk/article/ dear-white-men-need/1519321.
24 Bonnie Marcus (2018) 'Forget The Glass Ceiling. Female Attorneys Now Face A Concrete Wall', *Forbes*. Available at: www. forbes.com/sites/bonniemarcus/2018/06/15/forget-the-glass- ceiling-female-attorneys-now-face-a-concrete -wall/#338559da38f3.
25 Danielle Lee (2018) 'The Best Firms for Women: Building new networks of support', *Accounting Today*. Available at: www. accountingtoday.com/news/the-best-accounting-firms-for- women-building-new-networks-of-support.
26 Michelle Cheng, 'Why Minority Women Now Control Nearly Half of All Women-run Businnesses', *Inc*. Available at: www.inc. com/magazine/201811/michelle-cheng/minority-women-entre- preneur-founder-womenable.html.
27 Amanda MacMillan (2017) 'Can a Straight Woman Really Become a Lesbian Later in Life? The Truth About Sexual Fluidity', *Health*. Available at: https://www.health.com/condi- tion/sexual-health/sexual-fluidity.
28 Adrienne Rich (1980) 'Compulsory Heterosexuality and Lesbian Existence', *Signs*, 5(4), 631–660.
29 Stephanie Coontz (2020) 'How To Make Your Marriage Gayer', *New York Times*. Available at: https://www.nytimes.

com/2020/02/13/opinion/sunday/marriage-housework-gender
-happiness.html?referringSource=articleShare.

30 Garcia, M.A. and Umberson, D. (2019) 'Marital Strain and
Psychological Distress in Same-Sex and Different-Sex Couples'.
Fam Relat, 81: 1253–1268. doi:10.1111/jomf.12582.

31 Carlson, Daniel L., Hanson, Sarah, Fitzroy, Andrea (2016) 'The
Division of Child Care, Sexual Intimacy, and Relationship Quality
in Couples', *Gender & Society* 30(3):442–66.

32 Gupta, S. (1999) 'The Effects of Transitions in Marital Status on
Men's Performance of Housework', *Journal of Marriage and
Family*, 61(3), 700–711. doi:10.2307/353571.

33 Soraya Chemaly, *Rage Becomes Her* (London: Simon & Schuster,
2018) p.73.

34 Gaby Hinsliff (2019) 'The pansexual revolution: how sexual fluidity became mainstream', *Guardian*. Available at: www.theguard-
ian.com/society/2019/feb/14/the-pansexual-revolution-how-
sexual-fluidity-became-mainstream. The blog A Late Life
Lesbian Story is at https://alatelifelesbianstory.com.

35 Janice Turner (2019) 'Gary Lineker interview: on staying single
and battling Brexit', *The Times*. Available at: www.thetimes.
co.uk/article/gary-lineker-interview-on-staying-single-and-
battling-brexit-0z6kqqnss.

36 Live Population report. Available at: www.livepopulation.com/
country/united-kingdom.html.

37 Alyson Walsh (2020) 'I'm 56 and proud and here's what I know
about women in their 50s', That's Not My Age. Available at:
https://thatsnotmyage.com/health-wellbeing/im-56-and-proud
-and-heres-what-i-know-about-women-in-their-50s.

38 The Fashion Spot Diversity Report (2018).

39 Emma Hinchliffe (2020) 'Funding for female founders increased
in 2019 – but only to 2%', *Fortune*. Available at: https://fortune.
com/2020/03/02/female-founders-funding-2019.

40 Jeff Haden, 'A Study of 2.7 Million Startups Found the Ideal Age
to Start a Business (and It's Much Older Than You Think)', *Inc.*
Available at: https://www.inc.com/jeff-haden/a-study-of-27-
million-startups-found-ideal-age-to-start-a-business-and-its-
much-older-than-you-think.html.

41 Leslie Jamison (2018) 'I used to insist I didn't get angry. Not
anymore', *NYT*. Available at: https://www.nytimes.

com/2018/01/17/magazine/i-used-to-insist-i-didnt-get-angry
-not-anymore.html.

42 Quentin Fottrell (2019) `"Women are judged for being
emotional" - yet it's more acceptable for men to get upset and
angry, female executives say', *MarketWatch*.

43 Soraya Chemaly (2018) 'Why Women Don't Get to Be Angry',
Gen. Available at: https://gen.medium.com/rage-becomes-her
-why-women-dont-get-to-be-angry-b2496e9d679d.

44 Dale Vernor (2019) 'PTSD is more likely in women than men',
NAMI. Available at: https://nami.org/Blogs/NAMI-Blog/
October-2019/PTSD-is-More-Likely-in-Women-Than-Men.

SOURCES

Books

Benjamin, Marina, *The Middlepause* (London: Scribe, 2017)

Bushnell, Candace, *Is There Still Sex In The City?* (London: Little Brown, 2019)

Chemaly, Soraya, *Rage Becomes Her* (London: Simon & Schuster, 2018)

Connolly, Kieron, *Dark History of Hollywood.* (London: Amber Books, 2017)

D'Souza, Christa, *The Hot Topic* (London: Short Books, 2016)

De Maigret, Caroline, *Older But Better, But Older* (London: Ebury, 2020)

Diamond, Lisa, *Sexual Fluidity: Understanding Women's Love and Desire* (New York: Harvard University Press, 2009)

Doyle, Glennon, *Untamed* (London: Vermillion, 2020)

Greer, Germaine, *The Change* (London: Bloomsbury, 2018)

Hanauer, Cathi (ed), *The Bitch Is Back* (New York: HarperCollins, 2016)

Kreamer, Anne, *Going Gray* (New York: Little Brown, 2016)

Lewis, Jane, *Me and My Menopausal Vagina* (London: PAL Books, 2018)

Morgan, Eleanor, *Hormonal* (London: Virago, 2019)

Rubin, Gretchen, *The Four Tendencies* (London: Two Roads, 2017)

Steinke, Darcey, *Flash Count Diary* (London: Canongate, 2019)

Articles

Anderson, Gillian and Nadel, Jennifer (2017) 'The Truth is Out There (About Menopause)', *Lenny Letter*

Chemaly, Soraya (2018) 'Why Women Don't Get to Be Angry', *Gen*

Corcoran Harel, Monica (2020) 'Hollywood's Menopause Problem: "The Silence Around It Perpetuates Silence Among Women"', *Hollywood Reporter*

Devlin, Hannah (2020) 'Having more sex makes early menopause less likely', *Guardian*

Jamison, Leslie (2018) 'I used to insist I didn't get angry. Not anymore', *NYT*

Moore, Suzanne (2015) 'There Won't Be Blood', *New Statesman*

Oppenheim, Maya (2019) 'Menopausal women often prescribed antidepressants which make their symptoms worse, warn experts', *Independent*

Steinke, Darcey (2019) 'No One Told Me Exactly What to Expect From Menopause. But the Messages I Did Get Were Very Wrong', *Time*

Walsh, Alyson (2020) 'I'm 56 and proud and here's what I know about women in their 50s', That's Not My Age

Winterson, Jeanette (2014) 'Can You Stop the Menopause', *Guardian*

ACKNOWLEDGMENTS

As always there are dozens of people without whom this book would not be etc. etc. but none more so than my agent Abigail Bergstrom. Between Abi agreeing to represent me and the proposal for the book that became *The Shift* going out, my professional world went tits up. Throughout those dark months, Abi was stalwart, smart, insightful and calm. Her belief in me helped me regain belief in myself. It is no exaggeration to say that without her it would have taken me far longer to pick myself up and dust off the emotional debris. (And God knows it took long enough.) Thanks Abi. You are a legend. Scary, but a legend!

The other group who literally made this book happen are the coven of women who so kindly and candidly gave me their time, trust and the warts and all experiences that feature in the pages of this book. There are almost eighty of you in total - and many are identified only by first name, if at all, so I won't go and blow that by naming you all here – but you know who you are. I consider meeting and talking to you (mostly online – cheers lockdown) one of the greatest joys of writing this book. You made this book better just by sharing your stories. And I made a whole host of friends. Thank you. We will get together at some point, I promise.

Undying gratitude is also owed to Claire Mellon and Tessa Fane. If you've read the book, you'll know why. If not – why not?!

– in short, I'm not sure I would have been in any state to write this book without them.

Massive thanks also to my editor at Coronet, Hannah Black, who got it instantly and the wonderful team at Hodder (including but not limited to Veronique Norton, Erika Koljonen and Helen Flood) who have all championed *The Shift* from the moment it landed in their inbox. And the lawyer who made it publishable. And the design team! Never have I had a cover that has received so much love and adoration. I know we're not meant to judge books by their cover. But you know... we do. So thank you. And thanks to Megan Staunton and Rachel Quinn at Gleam for endless patience in the face of even more endless stupid questions. In fact, the whole Gleam family rocks.

On a personal note, I also owe unending gratitude to Marian Keyes and Damian Barr for their unwavering support and kindness in dark times. My not-so-little brother, And, and his wife, Al, who gave us a (rent-free) roof over our heads when we had sold our house but got locked down before we could move into the new one. My mum and dad who never quite know what hairbrained scheme I'm going to come up with next but always manage to come up smiling.

Jon. Always Jon. Thirty plus years of putting up with me, four months stuck in my brother's spare room in lockdown, 16 months trying to move house and somehow you're still speaking to me. Thank you. I love you.

And "little Sam", for hanging on in there, even when you thought you couldn't.